BETWEEN
HEAVEN
AND HELL

BETWEEN
HEAVEN
AND
HELL

THE STORY OF MY STROKE

DAVID TALBOT

CHRONICLE PRISM
SAN FRANCISCO

Text copyright © 2020 by David Talbot.

Library of Congress Cataloging-in-Publication Data available.

ISBN 978-1-4521-8333-6

Manufactured in Canada.

Interior design by Kelley Galbreath.

Typesetting by Cody Gates, Happenstance Type-O-Rama.

Cover design by Kelley Galbreath.

10 9 8 7 6 5 4 3 2 1

Chronicle books and gifts are available at special quantity discounts to corporations, professional associations, literacy programs, and other organizations. For details and discount information, please contact our premiums department at corporatesales@chroniclebooks.com or at 1-800-759-0190.

CHRONICLE PRISM

Chronicle Prism is an imprint of Chronicle Books LLC, 680 Second Street, San Francisco, California 94107

www.chronicleprism.com

*For Camille
and our enduring
circle of love*

"Be like the headland on which the waves continually break, but it stands firm and about it the boiling waters sink to sleep. Don't say, 'Unlucky am I, because this has befallen me.' Nay, rather: 'Lucky am I, because, though this befell me, I continue free from sorrow, neither crushed by the present, nor fearing what is to come.'"

MARCUS AURELIUS,
Meditations

CONTENTS

BETWEEN
HEAVEN
AND HELL

INTRODUCTION

On the evening of Friday, November 17, 2017, I began suffering a stroke while drinking and dining with friends at a restaurant in my longtime hometown, San Francisco. I write "began" because I was stricken by a "stuttering stroke," which took the next forty-eight hours to splutter to its conclusion. The stroke's onset was initially alarming, but soon became sufficiently clandestine for the first twenty hours or so to escape my concern. The initial odd feeling—a sort of darkening of my headlights—passed, and I shrugged it off, blaming one glass of wine too many. By the time the stroke had finished its damage, however, I found myself in the intensive care unit of a city hospital, with a small part of my brain dead from asphyxiation, and various mind and body functions severely disabled.

Lying in the hospital that would be my home for the next five weeks, my brain felt swirling and strangely muted at the same time. I was seeing double. The entire right side of my body—from the crown of my head to the toes on my foot—was partially paralyzed, and the limbs on that side of my body felt like dead weight. I couldn't get out of bed without nursing help. The left side of my face drooped and my speech was labored and barely understandable. My throat muscles were damaged and I could swallow only ice chips—one at a time, and with the greatest concentration, as nurses and loved ones nervously monitored me to make sure I didn't choke on or aspirate the bits of frozen water. I couldn't piss on my own and I had to be catheterized every few hours.

I was a fucking mess. And yet, I felt mysteriously elated. I was still alive—and I was still cognitively and physically intact enough for hospital authorities to decide after a two-day observation period that I passed their Darwinian survival test. This meant I could be transferred to the first-rate stroke ward at the Davies Campus of California Pacific Medical Center and begin to rebuild my life.

But my elation came not just from my medical good fortune, such as it was. I felt like I was being given another chance, not just to rebuild my life, but to restart it.

Before my stroke, at age sixty-six, I felt both encumbered and frantic. I had spent the past ten years or so shuttling back and forth to Hollywood, working with madcap directors and a revolving crew of producers and writers, in an endlessly vain effort to turn my history books into movies or TV series. I was driven by my family's chronic financial needs and by a desire, deep in my Hollywood bloodline, to see my work translated to the screen. My books *The Devil's Chessboard* and *Brothers* are dark explorations of the fraught relationship between American democracy and the national security state, including the shadowy labyrinth of the

Kennedy assassinations. Creative types in Hollywood found the books deeply alluring, yet terrifying to work on. The controversial projects inevitably attracted political intrigue and corporate back stories that I could barely fathom.

Stuck in the Hollywood morass and nearing the end of my career, I felt doubly mired. As a journalist and author and active participant in the historic convulsions of my times, I had experienced and accomplished most of what I wanted to in life—at least those things that were within my power. My wife, Camille, and I had nearly finished raising our two sons, Joe and Nat, and we had enjoyed and endured the mad ride of creating a family and holding on to it for dear life. For the first time in my memory, I felt that I was just kind of waiting around, that my heretofore hectic, overflowing life was coming to an end. And then it did.

As I sprawled in my hospital bed, feeling permanently dazed, I tried to describe what the experience felt like to my wife and sons through my slurred, labored speech. It felt, I said, like a cross between a brutal barroom beating and a spiritual awakening. I've spent my life rooted nearly exclusively in the joys and toils of the material world. At those times that I have felt transported to a higher realm, it has not been on the wings of angels. Instead I'd been soaring on love, music or a heady feeling that I'm part of some grand human movement to change the world. A more enlightened version of my generation's sex, drugs and rock 'n' roll mantra. But my stroke left me feeling exalted, in a way that I'd never felt before.

I felt more alive, and yet more in touch with death, than I had for a long time, maybe ever. I suppose I felt that I had died—because part of my brain literally had—and I'd come back to life.

It was like I was one of those mysterious middle-aged men you hear about now and then—men saddled with debts, overwork and family burdens who suddenly vanish into thin air, shedding the skin of their old lives and starting life anew somewhere as a different person.

At some point during my extended stay in the hospital, I began to realize that I liked this new me more than the old version. For one thing, he was physically braver. I used to be so phobic about intrusive medical procedures that I refused to have my blood drawn during visits to my doctor, to my great embarrassment. But after my stroke, I became so used to having needles jammed in my arms that I'd chat pleasantly with the lab technicians as they poked around looking for a promising vein. As nurses hovered over my groin with catheter tubes, wrestling to thread them expertly through my urethra, around the prostate gland and all the way to my bladder—a procedure that requires a miraculous amount of dexterity—I interviewed them about their lives in my journalistic style or listened to their stroke ward gossip.

That's another thing about this new person who was me—he was somehow more patient and attentive to others. Every person who came into my hospital room—neurologists, nurses, physical and occupational therapists, dietitians, psychology interns, religious counselors, stroke ward volunteers with comfort dogs for patients to pet, acupuncturists—seemed fascinating to me. Each of them was alive in the world, with a unique story to tell. Being a patient has taught me patience and empathy, and since my patient and outpatient care lasted for many months, I had time to absorb the lessons of my infirmity.

Most of all, my stroke reconnected me to my family. My head had been violently shaken free of emotional demons and manic work habits. My life was reduced to its essentials. I was so grateful I could still set eyes on my wife, sons, family and intimate friends—my circle of love—although it was through blurred vision. Thrown tightly together by urgent need, I soon rediscovered the precious joys of their company. The most comforting moments of my long hospital stay were the overnight vigils that Camille, Joe or Nat spent on a cot by my bedside, softly talking me to sleep and playing mixes of my favorite songs on the portable CD player they had brought to my room.

The old me always had an absurd, sometimes even dark, sense of humor. But after my stroke, I developed a heightened sense of how ridiculous and random life is—and how sublime. In my duress, I created a couple of alter egos. I would sometimes seek refuge in these split personalities when I felt emotionally overwhelmed. "Strokey" is a can-do kind of guy who can overcome any adversity in his way. "Nigel" is an endlessly sweet, wide-eyed chap who is torrentially appreciative of the slightest gesture of kindness. And for some reason he speaks in a charming English accent. At first, my family and friends were a bit puzzled by my new identities, but they've learned to accommodate them. When my wife wakes up next to me in bed some mornings, Nigel greets her with a cheery, "Aren't you *ever* so glad that I'm still breathing? I know that *I* certainly am!"

Also, I welcomed a new lighter me, as I shed nearly forty pounds, thanks initially to my difficulty swallowing, and then to the hospital's unappetizing menu and the nauseating side effects of my medication. By that point, adapting to a more

17

healthy diet did not seem like such a life-changing challenge. It simply felt like a way to enjoy life differently and to save my life. I don't recommend strokes as a diet plan, but there can be some gratifying physical repercussions. I no longer feel that I'm wearing my body, like an extra layer of heavy winter clothing. Despite my age, my flesh feels taut around my bones. I feel playful again in jeans and a T-shirt.

Finally, my stroke added another dimension to my writing. As a journalist and popular historian, my main obsession has been the world of power and politics. But for unsurprising reasons, my stroke has made me more introspective as a man and as a writer. These days, I'm deeply curious about the smaller details of daily life—like shopping and cooking—and about life's larger, inexplicable dimensions.

In the hospital, knowing I was a writer, the physical therapists soon began encouraging me to type again, even though the fingers on my right hand were excruciatingly clumsy and the words came out all garbled on the page. I thought these were futile exercises and that I would never write again. In my diminished state, even typing felt too daunting a task, let alone composing a paragraph or an entire essay. But coming back to life in a new way meant coming back to writing in a new way.

This book began on my Facebook page. I needed to make sense of what had happened to me, knowing that thousands of my invisible friends out there had suffered similar life-changing traumas, or loved someone who had. I needed to find out if I could still communicate and produce a response in others. I wanted to be educated and inspired—and even sometimes blown away—by those who knew all too well what I was going through.

I began tentatively posting this chronicle, "the story of my stroke," not long after returning home from the hospital, pecking awkwardly at my keyboard and having to correct every other word.

The responses from our weird, ethereal digital universe came instantly pouring in. Some were anguished cries about readers' own stricken brains and lives, some were beautifully crafted mini-masterpieces—philosophical musings about life's glory and suffering and ultimate meaning. These messages from the great beyond encouraged me to keep writing, to keep letting people inside my broken, changing life. And so I did, all during my first year of recovery, finally abandoning Facebook and writing for myself, until it became this book.

The novelist Rachel Cusk has observed that writing is "transmuted pain." And certainly writing this book has been emotionally cathartic for me. But I also hope to convey a sense of the strange joy that my stroke has bestowed on me. The sense of liberation from the dead weight of the past, or at least from those parts that have too much gravity. My stroke did not just change my life. It saved my life.

CHAPTER 1

BLOW-UP

T his is what it feels like to have a stroke. Or rather this is what my stroke felt like. Like Tolstoy's unhappy families, I've learned that each stroke is unhappy—or terrifying and hallucinatory—in its own way. Different strokes for different folks.

I was dining one fall evening with friends at an unassuming neighborhood French bistro. Nothing fancy, just a good roast chicken, green salad and chilled Chablis. The restaurant was mostly empty—ours was the most boisterous party, though we were few in number.

We were celebrating what seemed like an important step in the never-ending odyssey to turn my history books into Hollywood dramas. I think we were closing in on a top screenwriter, something like that. There've been so many twists and turns in this labyrinthine journey that I can't remember all the little happy endings, and unhappy setbacks, along the way.

Anyway, toasts were drunk to our ephemeral success, and as the meal concluded, I rose to my feet and instantly felt my life change. My mild sense of euphoria from the pleasure of the company and the smooth flow of wine . . . it all evaporated in a moment. I felt like the lights had dimmed, that I suddenly was dispatched to another dimension. And then I felt a curious sensation in the back of my head, like warm liquid rushing inside my skull. It was all very brief, and soon it seemed like the lights were fully turned back on. But I knew I'd just been transported somewhere I'd never been before, and I felt deeply unsettled.

———

My friends immediately noticed that something was wrong with me. "Are you OK?" asked one with a look of concern. But I assured them I felt fine—I had just stood up too quickly after the wine, I explained. In fact, I convinced them I was well enough to drive myself home. "Don't expire on us, we need you," joked one as I left to find my car. It somehow felt more ominous than funny.

Of course I should have stayed and admitted that I needed help. But as puzzling as it might sound, the truth is, I wanted to be alone. I didn't realize I was having a stroke; it felt instead as if something strange and special had just happened to me. Something more than just a wine-induced haze, something too intimate to share, even with close friends. I wanted to be inside myself; I wanted to figure out what was happening to me.

On the way home, I drove past Davies hospital on Castro Street, where I would be rushed in an ambulance thirty-six hours later. Yes, I should've pulled into the hospital driveway right then and checked myself into the intensive care unit. You can imagine how many times I dwelled on that missed turn later, when I lay in my hospital bed, hour after hour. What if, what if, what if . . . until I realized that mental fixation was a dead-end alley and if I kept going down it, I'd never find a way out.

But I include this information for all of you who might be fated to have strokes, or know and love someone who will. When I drove past Davies that night, I was still in the first hour of what would later be diagnosed as an ischemic stroke (a blocked blood vessel) that cut off the oxygen flow to my pons, a small area buried within the brain stem that controls such rather essential functions as breathing and heartbeat, as well as swallowing, speech, vision and coordination. Without a constant flow of oxygen, brain cells start dying at an alarmingly brisk speed—1.9 million per minute—so speedy treatment is essential.

If I had checked myself into the hospital within three hours of my first stroke symptoms, I might have been treated with a clot-dissolving drug known as tPA (tissue plasminogen activator). The clot-busting drug has its own hazards—it causes a fatal brain hemorrhage in about one in fifteen people. But I'll never know if my family and I would've played those odds because I didn't realize I was having a stroke until long after the three-hour window had closed.

I somehow drove home safely that night, enjoyed a sound sleep, and woke up the next morning full of my usual energy. I drove to the nearby Black Jet Bakery on Bernal Hill to buy almond croissants for my still slumbering family, then cooked for my brood the usual Saturday morning banquet of scrambled eggs, green onions and Jarlsberg cheese, accompanied by the platter of pastries. It was not until early evening, as I lay in bed reading, that my stroke clearly announced itself—nearly one full day after I had felt the lights flicker in my brain.

As I was reading, my vision suddenly blurred and my head felt like it was spinning. Just then my wife, Camille, arrived home after walking our dog, Brando, on the hill. I told her I couldn't see straight. I was gripped by the strong sensation that I was disappearing as we spoke, as those millions of brain cells went dark.

Camille immediately called my doctor's office and was told by the after-hours physician on call that I should go to a nearby walk-in clinic, those medical pop-ups you drop in on weekends when your doctor's office is closed. Wrong. At my age and with my history of high blood pressure, I should've been told to rush to the nearest emergency room.

Fortunately, or forebodingly, I began feeling so dire—dizzy, nauseated—in the car on the way to the weekend clinic that I told Camille I wouldn't make it there. So she quickly headed to the ER at St. Luke's, our neighborhood hospital, just a block away.

The medical tragicomedy continued at the St. Luke's emergency room, a grim holding pen in the bowels of the building. Because I was able to walk in, barely, the emergency staff didn't think I presented much of an emergency. While leisurely checking my vitals, the doctor examining me suggested I had a bad, if rather sudden and mysterious, case of the flu. Then, as he was about to release me, I began violently, explosively throwing up and the doctor changed his diagnosis.

"Let's get him upstairs," he said with a frown.

As I lay in the hospital room upstairs, my head swirling, I began to feel parts of my right side go numb. My head, neck, arm, hand, leg, foot, toes. A great heaviness was taking over that side of my body. I told my wife, who urgently relayed this news to the medical staff.

"It's probably just the potassium we're pumping in him," said a new, much younger doctor on weekend duty, airily dismissing my growing paralysis.

I was hauled onto a gurney and whisked down a long, bare hallway with dim lights to a remote tech room for a CT scan, to determine if bleeding was the cause of my crisis. It wasn't—the culprit was a clot. I should have also been given an MRI exam, which would have pinpointed the location and damage caused by my ischemic stroke. But the hospital staff informed Camille that it only had use of the MRI during weekdays. *Do they rent out the machine to other hospitals on Saturdays and Sundays*, she wondered?

By now, I felt my spirit beginning to waft from my body. As I was being wheeled down the shadowy hallway to the CT scan room, it seemed like a final passage of sorts. In fact, it felt oddly familiar—and then I recalled a similar image that I had used in my final Facebook post that afternoon. I used the photo of a murky hallway to illustrate a post about the dark times we live in. But, I wrote, we should take heart, quoting folk singer Jemima James's bittersweet song "Nothing New": "Long walk, dark hall, there's a door where there's a wall." Clearly, when I posted that message, my brain was already launched on some ineffable journey. I just didn't know it yet.

Inside the tight, tubular confines of the CT machine, I felt breathless and was gripped by panic for a moment. Then a great calm came over me. I felt powerless—as if the power to save myself was now beyond my control and I could only resign myself to my fate. I dozed off, and when I woke, I felt even more ethereal. I heard the technicians chatting and joking, like it was just another day in the office, which it was for them. One person's medical trauma is another person's night shift. But then I heard my oldest son, Joe—his angry, anxious voice cutting through the technicians' laughter, as he asked them to tell him what they were observing on their screen. Joe's voice was filled with worry and care, and it somehow tethered me back to this existence.

I slept fitfully in the hospital for a few hours that night. Whenever my mind swam upward toward consciousness, I felt like a stranger to myself. I could vaguely hear my wife speaking on her phone in a quiet, urgent voice to my sister Cindy, a doctor in Portland, Oregon. Cindy was able to diagnose my condition over the phone, based on what Camille was telling her—a clarity that was still eluding the St. Luke's medical team. "You've got to get him to the stroke ward at Davies hospital as quickly as you can," I later learned Cindy had told Camille.

Early that morning, when I fully awoke, my bed was surrounded by a half circle of hovering, familiar faces—Camille; our sons Joe and Nat; my brother, Steve; his wife, Pippa; and their daughter, Caitlin. This tableau of love and kindness reminded me of the last scene in *The Wizard of Oz*, when Dorothy wakes from her strange dream and is welcomed back by Aunt Em, Uncle Henry and the farmhands. Although Dorothy was coming back home, while I felt like I was making my final exit.

I began to say goodbye to my family. I thought it was important to tell them certain things while I still could. I told them I had lived the life I wanted to, and they shouldn't feel sad for me. I had no fear, and I wanted them to feel the same way. I was filled with love and serenity.

"You can't die." My wife's emphatic voice cut through my beatific surrender. "No, David—you just can't die."

And I understood in that moment that I couldn't give up yet. I might have lived the life I wanted, but others still needed me. And they weren't ready to let me go.

Life or death . . . it was still mostly out of my control. I was in the middle of what my doctor later called a "stuttering stroke." The brain trauma was pulsing, coming in waves, and it was still uncertain how badly damaged the progressing stroke would leave me. My mother and my aunt had suffered strokes at younger ages, long before me, and their attacks turned them into different people—fundamentally altering their personalities and intellects. The shocking transformations of these two vibrant women into diminished versions of themselves were twin shadows that hung over my extended family for years.

If I had any chance of living—and not having my identity erased—I needed to be transferred to the Davies stroke ward. By now my family had realized that St. Luke's seemed ill-equipped and not up to the task.[*] I heard Camille and other family members talking earnestly with the young St. Luke's

---

[*] Since my emergency medical ordeal, St. Luke's Hospital has been overhauled and relaunched as California Pacific Medical Center—Mission/Bernal Campus.

doctor, who was already in touch with the staff at Davies, and she assured my family that I would soon be transported there by ambulance.

But hours went by, and there was no ambulance. It was early Sunday morning, and there were unavoidable complications, my family was told. At one point, Camille was informed the ambulance was nearby, on the very same street as the hospital, in fact—but a half hour later it still hadn't arrived. I heard her becoming increasingly frustrated and angry with the hapless hospital staff.

Finally the ambulance crew arrived in a whoosh of urgency and efficiency. They smoothly bundled me onto a gurney and rolled me downstairs to the waiting vehicle. The three emergency technicians were my heroes. I had the feeling they were rescuing me from a sad medical ending. The air outside on the ER ramp was sharply cold. I knew by this point that I wanted to live. I started to thank the ambulance crew. But by now my speech was hopelessly sloppy. I couldn't make myself understood. Parts of me were still failing.

As we sped off, siren wailing, I could see San Francisco, the city that's been my life, flying by in the ambulance windows. The ambulance crew chief phoned the Davies ICU admissions team to alert them we were on the way. Fortune still seemed to be smiling on me, though like me, it had a crooked smile.

Suddenly there was tension in the crew chief's voice. "What do you mean there's no room? St. Luke's was supposed to set this up hours ago," he said into the phone, his tone rising.

The crew chief and the Davies administrator at the other end of the line argued for two or three minutes. My fate was in their hands. I began to laugh—the sound came out of my mouth like a strangled cry. I'm going to die because of a bureaucratic fuck-up. Somehow it seemed a properly absurd end.

But the ambulance chief would not be denied. "Look, I've got this guy en route, and I have nowhere else to take him. I'm bringing him to you. We'll be there in two minutes."

And that, dear readers, is how I made it into the tender, expert hands of the intensive care unit at Davies hospital. Because my wife simply refused to let me die. And because my ambulance crew chief was a stubborn, obstinate man who refused to take no for an answer.

Living, I learned that day, is sometimes a choice. And it takes effort—group effort.

The next morning I woke up in my bed in the Davies ICU, attached to softly purring machines. After my otherworldy weekend, the stroke was stuttering to its conclusion, and I began to assess the damage like a cleanup crew after a storm. My right arm and leg felt like dead weights, I was seeing double, I couldn't get out of bed on my own, and when I was helped to sit up, my head spun like a mad carousel. But damn, I had survived. I felt mangled, but oddly ecstatic, even celestial.

When I was a boy, I taught Sunday school and I was sent to an Episcopalian/military prep school (yes, odd combination). But since my boyhood, I've never felt religious. And though I was intrigued by all the spiritual movements of my 1960s youth, particularly when the Beatles made their famous sojourn to India, I've never devoted myself to a spiritual regimen. So the sudden flowering of my mind took me by surprise as I regained consciousness.

I later learned that Ram Dass—whose legendary journey had taken him from Harvard psychology professor to LSD pioneer to Maharaji devotee to baby boom generation guru— had suffered a stroke at sixty-six, the same age when my mind was blown. But ironically he did not experience his trauma in spiritual terms. Eventually, Ram Dass later observed, his stroke imbued him with a "fierce grace," bringing him closer to God. But while in its initial grip, he felt nothing heavenly—which made him feel like he "had a lot more spiritual work to do."

For whatever reason, my stroke brought this supremely Earth-bound man closer to some kind of transcendence. I was amazed by its mind-opening power on me—by, yes, its fierce grace.

After a typhoon blows through your brain and your life, and you are washed up onshore more dead than alive, you have to decide how you're going to proceed with the time remaining to you on Earth. Suddenly you've been left halfway between heaven and hell. I was determined to live the rest of my life closer to heaven.

CHAPTER 2

HOLLYWOOD GAVE
ME A STROKE

Hollywood gave me a stroke. Not literally, of course. There were other factors: weight, blood pressure, genetics. But I remember with utter clarity the afternoon meeting in a top Hollywood director's office—just weeks before my actual stroke—when I felt my head was going to explode.

It was the latest in a series of show business meetings to discuss how to turn my 2015 book, *The Devil's Chessboard,* into a dramatic TV series. I felt that my epic history of the CIA spymaster Allen Dulles and the rise of America's powerful national security labyrinth was the culmination of my career as a popular historian. Though it was a dark and dense saga—featuring many characters and global events from FDR's New Deal era to JFK's New Frontier—I had tried to write the book as a gripping spy drama. So I was pleased that reviewers appreciated its narrative drive, with the *Daily Beast* book critic declaring that "neither [John] le Carré nor Graham Greene could do any better."

But the mainstream press had found *The Devil's Chessboard* too alarming to even review, with my conclusion that Dulles and his clandestine circle had organized the assassination of President Kennedy and its cover-up. An editor at the *Washington Post* flatly told my book publicist, "We're not going to touch this one with a ten-foot pole." Despite the corporate media blackout, my book still became a *New York Times* bestseller.

To its credit, the *Washington Post* more recently has demonstrated a willingness to open the long-sealed doors to the assassinations of both President Kennedy and his brother Senator Robert F. Kennedy. As for Hollywood, the entertainment capital has long been tantalized but deeply wary of the shadowy subject.

On that fateful afternoon, a full cast was assembled in the director's office, including the A-list filmmaker himself, various assistants, producers, consultants and premier TV writers whom he had summoned (one via Skype from New York), along with my book research colleague and close friend, Karen Croft, and me.

These meetings, which had been going on and off for several months, had a strange life of their own, in that Hollywood way, and never seemed to reach any conclusive destination. That afternoon, we leaped about wildly through my sprawling espionage chronicle, which featured Nazi spies, Wall Street collaborators, Washington power brokers, Strangelovian Cold War characters—and the idealistic leaders, political pawns, wives and mistresses who fell before these global chess masters. Story ideas, psychological observations and other random epiphanies were hurled at the walls, but nothing seemed to stick.

Now and then, the exasperated director would impatiently call on me to provide yet another synopsis of my six-hundred-page book. I felt that I had to translate the tome I considered my life's greatest work into television terms that the group could easily grasp. In bursts of twenty words or less.

I felt under mounting pressure to deliver creatively that day—despite my lack of television experience—for financial reasons. Book writing is no way to support a family, so of course Hollywood looms as the golden ring for authors. The money at this stage of the consulting process was minimal, but if by some miracle *The Devil's Chessboard* went into production and found a big enough TV audience, perhaps I'd never again have to lose sleep over my family's financial future.

So I was trying my hardest to make this meeting in the director's office succeed. I recalled other chaotic meetings in my journalism days, when I was running the online publishing start-up *Salon*, and my staff and I were wildly brainstorming about the week's news and how to cover it in a unique and brave way. But those meetings, as freewheeling as they were, had more logic—they almost always produced something good and tangible.

In the director's office, I felt completely frustrated and bewildered. Deep down, in the midst of all the verbal commotion, I knew this meeting would result in nothing. I had come to believe that my friend Oliver Stone was right when he told me, "Your books will never be made in Hollywood—they're too afraid of them." Oliver had already been through the firestorm of *JFK* (1991)—he knew the system wasn't going to allow something like that again. Even before Oliver finished filming his powerful dramatic interpretation of the Kennedy assassination, his script was leaked to the press and he was widely pilloried as a "conspiracy freak" and worse. The smears stuck to the director for years, despite his film's box office success. The public uproar over *JFK* pressured Congress into passing the President John F. Kennedy Assassination Records Collection Act of 1992. Thousands of government documents related to the Kennedy presidency and assassination were released under this law, but the CIA still withholds many relevant documents to this very day, in blatant defiance of Congress.

This clammy fever still grips the Kennedy story in Hollywood. In fact, one of the TV writers who greeted me that afternoon in the director's office asked me with a nervous chuckle, "Why aren't you dead?" He was referring to my book's exploration of the CIA's dark catacombs.

Despite it all, my desire to be financially saved by Hollywood was too strong—and so I flailed around at the meeting, trying to verbally transform my book into the next big spy thriller through sheer willpower. About two hours into the marathon meeting, my head started pounding and expanding. I felt dizzy and frantic at the same time. I could feel my blood pressure—which despite years of daily medication was still chronically high—spiking dangerously. I knew I had to get out of the room, and I excused myself to go to the bathroom, leaving it to Karen to keep dramatizing our book.

In the bathroom down the hall, I splashed water on my face and tried to slow the galloping pulse in my chest and head. I steadied myself against the sink in case I passed out. I knew I shouldn't return to the meeting. But minutes later, I did. Doing so, I sealed my fate.

It wasn't just the promise of a big payday. Hollywood is literally in my blood. My parents were a showbiz couple. They first "met" at New York's Radio City Music Hall, where my mother, Paula, came as a girl from her family home in New Jersey to watch movies. It was there that she first saw my handsome Black Irish father, Lyle, who loomed over her on the screen (and soon in her dreams). My mother embarked on her own show business career while still a teenager, singing at military bases for troops on their way to World War II, and then heading to Hollywood, where she began acting in theater to get experience and studio attention. Her movie fan dreams came true when she shared a stage with my father, then his bed (despite their twenty-six-year age gap), and then ran off with him to Tijuana to get married.

The marriage—my father's fifth—should never have worked. And it sometimes didn't. But they were held together by a palpably erotic bond. It seemed that both of them couldn't believe their good luck—the aging actor with a declining career finally finds the love of his life in the form of a nineteen-year-old busty blonde beauty, who was not only an aspiring actress-singer but the daughter of two brainy educators and the sister of a rocket scientist. And my mother got the man of her screen dreams, then worked so hard on him and with him that she made him something real: a surprisingly good husband and father.

Hollywood suffused our family home when my three siblings and I were growing up—it was the other bond that held my parents together. They were constantly swapping show business shoptalk in the kitchen or over dinner. Gossip about "the business" and the ups and downs of fellow actors was our family's lingua franca. All six of us were so excited at Academy

Awards time as we gathered around our TV console that it felt as though *we* were nominated for Oscars.

On special Saturday afternoons, Paula would whisk us off to a Hollywood movie theater that played film classics whenever one of her all-time favorites, like *Wuthering Heights,* was being shown. We would sit in the audience surrounded by older gay men who knew their film history and aging sirens who looked like they might once upon a time have acted with Merle Oberon. After these film screenings, our mother would regale us with ageless dish about the stars we'd just seen as if she knew them.

So I've loved Hollywood madly ever since I was a kid, since I choked back tears as Heathcliff carried Cathy to the window for one last look at their beloved heather-covered hills. Of course, Hollywood mythology and reality are two different things. The business behind the screen can be the most sleazy and brutal that America has to offer. Words don't mean anything—the more praise I would hear about my books, the more I knew they didn't have a chance.

Actually, my frustrating Hollywood journey had begun a decade earlier, with the publication of my first history book, *Brothers: The Hidden History of the Kennedy Years.* During one meeting about *Brothers* at Starz, the cable network's deeply tanned TV chief, Chris Albrecht, who entered the room in shoes that seemed meant to elevate his height, kept boasting he had the guts to make my book the "tentpole" series for his new season. Like *The Devil's Chessboard, Brothers* tapped into America's troubled dreams about Kennedy's Camelot, telling the story of Robert Kennedy's secret search for the truth about his brother's assassination. Of course, it turned out that

Albrecht had no courage to tackle such a story. His office called just days later to say no go.

I later learned that Albrecht had an ugly past. He had ended up at the lower budget cable channel Starz after being forced to resign by the more prestigious network HBO for assaulting his girlfriend outside a Las Vegas boxing match. Nowadays these stories of rampant abuse and outrageous behavior are everywhere. What is not as widely discussed is the sheer madness of the Hollywood creative process itself. Where story meetings have all the clarity of a Mad Hatter tea party and some king or queen is constantly screaming, "Off with your head, off with your head!"—until, sure enough, it finally blows sky-high like a Champagne cork.

Since my stroke, I've kept my distance from the Hollywood wonderland. I can't give up my dreams entirely because it's, well, the dream factory, and dreams die hard. But since I want to live, I communicate with Hollywood's mad hatters through intermediaries. I try not to take anything industry-related too seriously, even when I'm told that my books might serve as the basis for a new James Bond franchise. "Fantastic!" I say with the kind of false conviction and enthusiasm I learned in Hollywood.

Still, I haven't grown entirely cynical about the entertainment world where I grew up. Some movies and TV shows still manage to make me feel like I'm in that old Hollywood movie theater with my mother, bathed in a dream light. My oldest son, Joe, also became infected with this dark magic somewhere along the way, and in early 2018 he began directing his first feature film, *The Last Black Man in San Francisco*. Whenever I worry about what he will encounter in his future, I remind myself that he doesn't have to follow my same path. For one thing, he's a director and enjoys a much higher status in the Hollywood food chain than lowly authors.

I hope that my frustrating Hollywood experience, which continues to this day, can also be educational for Joe. I pray that his old man's volatile temperament—and yes, my stroke—serve as cautionary lessons for him.

One afternoon I watched my son directing an emotionally difficult scene on film location in a gingerbread San Francisco mansion. Dozens of film crew workers raced here and there getting ready for the shot, while the actors brooded intensely as they slipped into character. The atmosphere was fraught and frantic. I was getting nervous for Joe. But there he was, in the eye of the storm, quietly conferring with the cinematographer. How had he learned to be so centered, so calmly in command? On the set of his very first feature-length movie?

If I want to have a longer life, I need to learn from Joe too.

CHAPTER 3

RIDING THE DRAGON

My high-stress career actually began years before my Hollywood mad carnival. It started back in 1995, when I launched *Salon*, one of America's first online publications, at the dawn of the wild dot-com roller-coaster ride. I could easily have suffered a stroke or heart attack anytime during the ten years I served as *Salon's* editor in chief and chairman of the board—a dual editorial/business role that allowed me to protect the journalistic integrity of my creation but unfortunately subjected me to all the joys and horrors of that brave new digital era.

At some point in a high-anxiety career, you have to ask yourself, "Am I prepared to die for this? Is this truly worth my life?" Because even though you might deny this awful truth for some time, eventually you will have to answer the question. It's a life or death question that—depending on how you answer it—can make your mark on the world . . . and can kill you.

This stark truth hit me one afternoon in fall 1998 while at my desk in the corner office of *Salon,* which at the time occupied a former art gallery above the Rochester Big and Tall men's clothing store in downtown San Francisco. I was anxiously awaiting a business visit from John Warnock, co-founder of the software giant Adobe and the biggest investor in *Salon.* Warnock was a courteous middle-aged man with a professorial beard and a thoughtful manner to match. He was not a typical, robotic Silicon Valley engineering mogul. He had clearly invested millions of his own money in *Salon* not strictly as a business venture, but because he also cared about free speech and the future of American journalism. But Warnock was still a businessman. And he had the power of life and death over my shaky start-up, which like all dot-com publishing ventures was still struggling to find a stable business model after three wild years in operation.

About an hour before Warnock was due to arrive, I swallowed a pill that my doctor had prescribed to help me quell my galloping anxieties. I had tried one or two other medications at the time to calm my nerves and help me sleep at night, but none of them made much difference. This one did—in an emphatic way. I passed out at my desk, waking moments later with a racing heart and a profound sense of disorientation.

Flushed and sweating, I walked in a daze through the field of cubicles that jammed our office, heading for the rooms of my two top editorial colleagues, Andrew Ross and Gary Kamiya. I remember the faces of the young *Salon* employees who all looked up at me as I went rushing by, which they usually did, searching for some sign of how the company was faring by the either giddy or anguished look on my face. This was not a good time to be making eye contact with me—Daddy looked like a wreck.

————

Bursting in on a news meeting between Ross and Kamiya—my longtime friends and journalistic partners—I announced in a strangled voice that I thought I was having a heart attack. They looked as stricken as I felt. They quickly called for an ambulance, even though I knew the timing was terrible. What about Warnock? The future of *Salon*'s funding depended on a smooth business meeting—a meeting scheduled to begin in just minutes. But my life was apparently at stake. As we were waiting for the ambulance, I felt I might lose consciousness at any moment and I breathlessly begged Gary to look out for Camille and our two young boys. Then we heard the ambulance, with sirens wailing, screech to a halt outside the building.

As two burly emergency medical technicians strapped me onto a gurney and prepared to wheel me to the elevator, Andrew announced that Warnock had arrived in the downstairs lobby. "Wait!" I hissed at the ambulance crew. "You can't take me down in the elevator." Even though I thought I was dying, I couldn't bear the idea of *Salon*'s crucial financial supporter seeing the company founder being hauled out of the building on a stretcher. I might or might not actually expire, but I knew that eye-popping visual would definitely kill *Salon*.

I demanded to be released from the gurney and allowed to walk down the back stairwell, to avoid bumping into Warnock.

The medics were aghast—my blood pressure was soaring and I could die right there. They made me agree to sign a legal release before they unstrapped me.

I made it downstairs with the medics nervously at my side, and as I was raced to a nearby hospital, Andrew and Gary, along with *Salon* CEO Michael O'Donnell, were left to explain to Warnock my strange absence from the crucial meeting. They put on a brilliant show in my absence and fortunately, Warnock was persuaded to save *Salon* by leading another round of investment.

Meanwhile, I found myself in the emergency room of St. Francis Hospital, plugged into an electrocardiogram machine. "Are you in a stressful line of work?" the ER doctor asked me. He could see that my heart was fine, but that I was probably in the throes of a massive anxiety attack, triggered by the pill I had popped and many months of unrelieved work pressure. "You could say that," I replied. "I run a dot-com start-up."

"Yeah, we see a lot of you guys in here," said the doctor.

I could have talked to the doctor for a full hour about all the pressures that were compounding in my life. And I was only three years into my frenzied run at *Salon*. My frantic stairwell exit should have been a cautionary siren for me. Instead it would become a funny barroom anecdote, another *Salon* near-death experience.

Fall 1998 was full of such madcap terror. That September *Salon* broke the most explosive story in its history, an exposé of Representative Henry Hyde's five-year sexual affair with a married woman. Headlined "This hypocrite broke up my family," the cover story told of the powerful Republican congressman's adulterous affair from the aggrieved point of view of the woman's ex-husband. What made the tawdry story newsworthy, from my perspective, was that Hyde—as the family-values champion who chaired the House Judiciary Committee—was about to preside over a Congressional inquiry to decide whether President Bill Clinton should be impeached for his own illicit affair. The hypocrisy, as the man cuckolded by Hyde bitterly pointed out to *Salon*, was rank.

As soon as we pushed the button on the Hyde story, all hell broke loose. America was just plunging into the political civil war that would continue to rage hotter and hotter, and our little news engine had sprayed oil on the fire. I was suddenly dragged into the center of the media glare, forced to defend *Salon*'s publishing decision on TV shows ranging from Bill O'Reilly's Fox News fight cage to a George Stephanopoulos ABC News program. Surprisingly, Stephanopoulos expressed even more outrage over *Salon*'s exposé than O'Reilly did. As Clinton's former communications director, he was apparently trying to prove that he was now willing to toe the corporate news line and attack his former boss.

In fact, *Salon*'s investigative reporting and commentary on the Clinton impeachment circus—led by Murray Waas and Joe Conason—sharply separated our publication from the mainstream media. While the rest of the press pack obsessively and salaciously focused on Monica Lewinsky's stained dress and Clinton's other "bimbo eruptions," *Salon* published a stream of exclusives on the deeply partisan operation of special prosecutor Kenneth Starr and the "vast right-wing conspiracy" behind it (in Hillary Clinton's words).

Salon was not particularly fond of Clinton's presidency, which we found too centrist and Wall Street–cozy. But, unlike nearly the entire Washington press corps, we didn't feel that he should be impeached for sexual acts that we concluded at the time were sleazy but consensual. (The rise of the #MeToo movement in later years would shine a harsher light on Clinton's personal abuse of power.) And the Republican opposition spearheaded by House Speaker Newt Gingrich (who was guilty of his own flagrant moral hypocrisy) that was trying to overthrow Clinton would have been disastrous for the country.

Already resented by the mainstream press for our ink-and-paper-threatening digital innovation, *Salon* now found itself doubly isolated and alone because of our Clinton coverage. I was watching CNN on my bedroom TV while dressing for work one morning when I saw Texas congressman Tom DeLay, Gingrich's viperish henchman, call for the FBI to investigate *Salon* for obstructing the impeachment process. Conservative attack groups organized a boycott of *Salon* advertisers. A *Wall Street Journal* editorial pilloried our leading investors by name. Our office was hit by perhaps the first politically motivated "denial of service" e-mail blackout attack. At the same time, in what was clearly a coordinated maneuver, our office received an all-too-credible bomb threat, which sent not only our own staff rushing to the exits, but the occupants of the entire building. I remember the building manager glaring at me in the office parking lot, where we all huddled as the high-rise was swept by a security team. Her furious expression said it all: *I knew I shouldn't have rented to you people.*

The political firestorm further threatened *Salon*'s already tenuous existence, but it also had the opposite effect of suddenly inflating our readership. Thousands of people, tired of the media's one-dimensional coverage of the Clinton crisis, flocked to *Salon* to read our deep reporting on the Republican impeachment juggernaut. I internalized each stomach-churning dive and rise in *Salon's* roller-coaster fortunes, despairing of our survival one day and rejoicing at the meteoric surge of our circulation the next.

Salon's new notoriety began winning attention from big media brands, including Time Warner and the *New York Times*, which began courting us for a potential acquisition. And other rising digital companies loomed as potential partners. Hearing about a promising new search engine start-up being incubated near the Stanford campus, my always enterprising business wingman, *Salon* CEO O'Donnell, headed down the peninsula one afternoon to see if he could buy the new venture, which its two young founders were calling Google. Mike was a former quarterback for UC-Berkeley's Golden Bears and he was always looking for the next big opening. O'Donnell found Google's young creators, Larry Page and Sergey Brin, in a modest Menlo Park ranch house, where they were hatching their start-up, not far from the Stanford dorms where they were still living. Because of all the buzz that *Salon* was getting at the time, one of Google's inventors—Page—seemed intrigued by O'Donnell's acquisition offer. But co-founder Brin was dismissive. "Are you kidding?" he sneered. "We're going to be worth a billion dollars someday." Brin seriously undervalued Google's future worth—as I write this, its parent company, Alphabet, is hovering around the $740 billion mark.

As the top "creative" executive at *Salon,* I was often called on to participate in these high-stakes business meetings, where

45

our future direction and identity were always on the table. It was my job to explain *Salon*'s vision and to see if the partnership could take both companies to a new level.

So one day I found myself sitting with O'Donnell and our marketing vice president, Marc Wernick, in a conference room at the Amazon headquarters in Seattle. Our executive team had been brainstorming with Amazon's business development team for weeks, exploring how *Salon* could connect its robust book review department to Amazon's e-commerce engine—an editorial-sales linkage that was innovative at the time. The Amazon managers seemed confident they had done due diligence on the deal and they just needed the final sign-off from their boss, Amazon founder Jeff Bezos.

———

A few minutes into our meeting, Bezos himself came bounding into the room. He was pulsing with energy and was obviously pressed for time. That's my memory of my ten frenetic years at *Salon*—time was money and each slot on the business calendar could make or break my beloved little company.

"So how's this deal supposed to work?" asked Bezos, cutting to the chase. As the Amazon biz development chief began explaining the proposed partnership, he sounded nervous, with a slight quiver to his voice—a man who had seemed so suave and self-assured in our earlier meetings. He described how *Salon* readers would be directed to Amazon to buy the books that were reviewed by our critics; in return Amazon would link to *Salon* so book buyers could explore our deep literary coverage.

Bezos abruptly cut him off and laser-stared at me and my *Salon* colleagues. "Let me get this straight," he said, his voice rising. "You want me to send my big pipeline of customers to your site?"

Well, yeah, we said, as his underlings—who clearly had experienced their boss's mercurial behavior before—looked nervously down at the floor.

"I might as well stick a gun in my mouth and blow my fucking head off!" Bezos erupted. He mimed sticking the barrel of the gun in his mouth for added emphasis.

Awkward silence. But moments later, after some further discussion of how the deal could work to Amazon's benefit and not just *Salon*'s, Bezos had a sudden change of heart. He offered to buy *Salon*. "What are you worth?" he asked. From rejected suitor to bride in a flash!

We probably should've immediately taken the deal, because the *Salon* executive team would all be flush with Amazon stock today. But each one of these white-knuckle meetings with the new masters of digital capitalism or with the captains of traditional media was not just a test of our business acumen. It was a sort of moral crucible for me, testing my commitment to aggressive, independent journalism. The golden dot-com treasure always seemed to be dangling within our outstretched reach at *Salon*, but it always came with a price. Did I really want to be working under a temperamental, unpredictable business genius like Bezos? I had started *Salon* to be free of such corporate madness. How would operating as an Amazon subsidiary curtail our editorial independence? And how would my staff—whose morale and well-being I was always thinking of—fare under such a merger?

Salon was my dream come true, a journalistic playhouse where the editors and reporters were fully in control. The "suits"— investors, advertisers and competing media executives—had not yet figured out the web as a publishing medium so we were free to experiment, take creative risks and invent online journalism as we went along. It was important to me that we were based in free-spirited San Francisco, where we defied New York's insular media establishment, building our pioneering digital publication around the liberated voices of the West Coast and with the rocket boost of investment capital from Silicon Valley. No publication with as strangely refreshing an editorial mix could have gone into business in corporate New York—or in slick Los Angeles, for that matter.

Salon combined independent political reporting and investigative journalism with sophisticated cultural coverage, bawdy sex and celebrity coverage, and wicked humor. I called it a "smart tabloid"—and it became the template for a later wave of online magazines, none of which captured *Salon*'s peculiar Left Coast alchemy. In conceptualizing *Salon*, I drew on my love for earlier San Francisco upstart publications, including *Ramparts* magazine under the madcap genius and radicalism of editors Warren Hinckle and Robert Scheer, and Jann Wenner's pre-New York *Rolling Stone*, in the era of Hunter Thompson's gonzo journalism.

Like all breakthrough publications, *Salon* gave an early, national platform to bold up-and-coming writers who helped define our iconoclastic identity. We featured such rising original voices as contributors Camille Paglia, Dave Eggers, Glenn Greenwald, David Sedaris, Sarah Vowell, Anne Lamott,

Augusten Burroughs, Sallie Tisdale and Max Blumenthal, as well as staff members like Laura Miller, Dwight Garner, Jake Tapper, Joan Walsh, Gary Kamiya, Stephanie Zacharek, Michelle Goldberg, Rebecca Traister, Carina Chocano, D. Watkins and Steve Kornacki—who were all headed for a bigger media stage.

By featuring a unique package of original reporting and colorful writing, *Salon* was able to sell subscriptions to our readers, something very rare on the internet. At our height we attracted nearly 100,000 paid readers, who each shelled out $40 a year for "Salon Premium." This total of nearly $4 million in annual revenue accounted for half our budget—the rest we tried to scrape together by selling advertising, always a challenge in an ad market dominated by tech giants like Google and Yahoo.

Despite our respectable (if erratic) revenue stream, *Salon* was always on the verge of bankruptcy because we were building a good-sized newsroom and we believed in paying staffers and freelancers decent money. Speedy growth and market share were the mantras of dot-com capitalism—it was a frantic online land grab, and the start-ups that could accumulate the most user bandwidth and establish the biggest brand names the fastest were going to be the new medium's winners. So even after *Salon* raised $25 million in its 1999 initial public offering (IPO), we were soon low on cash again.

At the elite digital business summits to which I began to be invited, all the young masters of the new media universe kept voicing the hypergrowth mantra, even at the cost of running their companies at terrifying burn rates. CNET founder Halsey Minor—a tall, handsome WASP who seemed to step out of a

Ralph Lauren ad—had a cocky expression at the time: "You die hitting the wall at forty or one hundred, so you might as well drive one hundred." To this day, I don't know whether we were driving *Salon* too fast or not fast enough.

In any case, I loved the rush and the heady sense that we were leaving the old, slow corporate media in the dust. "Right here, right now / there is no other place I want to be," as the British alt-rock band Jesus Jones sang in the '90s. That's how I felt at *Salon*—right in the middle of the new media revolution as the world woke up "from history."

That's why I felt it was all worth it, even if I keeled over in my office and died from stress overload way before my time. How many journalists can say they truly made a difference, that they not only changed their profession—if only for a brief and shining moment—but affected the course of national affairs?

In the middle of the Clinton impeachment circus, I was invited to a gathering at the White House with my *Salon* comrades Kamiya and Ross to meet with the president. Clinton was obviously intrigued by this little West Coast media upstart that kept breaking stories about the Republican impeachment machine. "*Salon*," he would later tell confidants, "saved my ass." Clinton grilled us about our reporting and finances—smart questions that revealed how much he already knew about the emerging online new medium. I remember how tired he looked in the midst of the endless crisis, with big bags under his eyes. In fact, Clinton spoke directly about his fatigue at one point, recalling how President Lyndon Johnson also found it hard to sleep in the White House as the Vietnam War deteriorated. "Sleeping badly can cause you to make bad decisions," Clinton observed.

Hillary Clinton also joined us in the Diplomatic Reception Room, where Franklin Roosevelt had delivered his legendary fireside chats. She too seemed emotionally drained and bunkered in a way that felt weirdly familiar to me. But I remember thinking that Hillary was every bit as shrewdly combative as her husband. She shared a fascinating story with us: "You know, when we began talking about Bill running for president, we got a call from Boyden Gray," who was then a White House counsel for President George H. W. Bush, and a longtime *consigliere* in Bush's preppy mafia. "He told us that Bill had a bright political future ahead of him and if he waited another four years to run, they wouldn't stand in his way—in fact they'd make it easy for him. But if he ran against Bush in '92, they'd destroy him. I said, 'Bill, what do you think they mean?' Now we know."

The Clintons decided to plunge forward despite the scorching animosity and exposure that awaited them. What sort of courage, or hubris, does that take? In my much smaller way, I had made the same bargain by starting *Salon* and leading it into the country's political maelstrom. What complicated my brash decision was the fact that I was a family man, and Camille was deeply ambivalent about my career trajectory—even though she too was a *Salon* editor, launching the groundbreaking "Mothers Who Think" satellite site with novelist Kate Moses. Meanwhile our two young sons had no say at all about their father's risky professional path.

While I was embroiled in the Washington madness, right-wing attack dogs began personally targeting me. I received death threats over my home phone. A conservative reporter approached an ex-girlfriend and asked if she could give him any dirt on me, making it clear that his magazine would reward her. The *Salon* strains on our marriage pushed it to the breaking point and Camille and I began seeing a therapist named Lillian Rubin, a sharply intuitive analyst of family life known for her bestselling books *Worlds of Pain* and *Intimate Strangers*. These marriage counseling sessions are a blur to me now, because I sandwiched them in between a stack of business appointments. But after my stroke, Camille reminded me of what Rubin advised me years ago.

Rubin understood the pressures I was under at *Salon*, and she sympathized with our journalistic mission. In fact she wrote occasionally for the publication. But she told me that I was not the only stressed-out executive among her clients—she had another walking time-bomb, and he could only change his life after he had a heart attack. "Now when he flies off to some city for an important business meeting," Rubin said, "he always makes time to go to a museum or an art gallery or take a walk in the park."

As I said, I can't remember Rubin giving me this warning. But even if it had sunk in at the time, I doubt it would have made a difference. I believed then that *Salon* was worth dying for. We were caught up in history's hurricane. And I couldn't see any way to buffer myself from the storm without seriously jeopardizing *Salon*'s chances for success. I was convinced that surviving in the Darwinian dot-com world required reckless courage.

I deeply loved my family, but I also believed that I had an extended family and I needed to care for the growing staff at *Salon*, which expanded at its peak to well over one hundred people. Many of them made sacrifices to work at *Salon* because they believed in me and in our editorial crusade. They struggled under the same financial, personal and political pressures.

In any event, I was spared a fateful reckoning while riding the dragon at *Salon*. That would come years later.

CHAPTER 4

ALIVE AGAIN: LIFE ON THE STROKE WARD

I spent five weeks in the Davies hospital stroke ward—five harrowing, hallucinatory and surprisingly hallowed weeks that still haunt me. I'll never forget my confinement there— even now when I tell stories to friends about my long hospitalization, I feel like I'm being transported back to that strange middle world, suspended between life and death.

But the truth is, I don't want to forget what I went through on the stroke floor because it changed me in ways I never want to fade. Near death on arrival at the hospital, I was forced to call upon inner resources never before tested so severely, and to depend on the skills and compassion of a circle of complete strangers for my survival. I needed to be more heroic—and, at the same time, more trusting of others—than at any other moment in my life. It's vital that you remind everyone around you at the hospital that you're still a human being, even when you feel like a gravely wounded animal. The hospital care providers were not my family, but I soon realized that I needed them to care about me as if we were connected by blood.

I spent the first nights of my hospitalization in the Davies intensive care unit, but my family and I knew that my ultimate destination must be the second-floor stroke ward, which was nationally renowned for the high quality of its care. After observing the progress of my stroke over a forty-eight-hour period, the medical staff decided I was still mentally and physically intact enough to qualify for rehabilitation. (Those too badly damaged by their strokes were destined to be warehoused in some long-term care facility for hopeless cases—a fate that unfortunately awaited the member of a well-known indie rock band in the ICU room next to mine.) But when I was ready to be transferred, there were no empty beds on the coveted stroke floor, so before entering heaven, I had to be temporarily shelved in a third-floor purgatory, which housed the full spectrum of human casualties.

This turned out to be the bleakest stretch of my lengthy hospital confinement. The long nights on this dreary hospital floor were frequently punctured by the shrieking and wailing of dementia patients. "Somebody help me! Oh God, help me! Why won't anyone help me!" Even though the harried nursing staff kept rushing to their bedsides to reassure them, the distraught patients couldn't let go of their demons. Actually, the two nights on that floor were more hell than purgatory. I didn't know where the other patients' anguish left off and mine began.

The nurse who was supposed to be attending me at nights was so frazzled by the screaming patients that on the rare occasions he did show up at my bedside to administer medications, his hands were shaking. He was so distracted by the tormented patients, who kept struggling to get out of their beds, that he neglected to empty my catheter bag on time, with unfortunate results for me.

Even sadder to me than the dementia patients was the man who shared my room. He had been admitted some time before me, when a neighbor discovered him wasting away from malnutrition in his apartment. One morning a social worker came to visit with him, because my roommate had gained some weight in the hospital and was about to be discharged.

"Is there anyone who can pick you up and take you home?" she asked.

No, he softly replied, there was no one.

"What about the neighbor who called for help when he found you?" she asked.

Well, we used to be friends, said the man, but not anymore.

"How about family? You wrote down the name of a niece when you were admitted."

She lives in Cleveland, explained the man, and I haven't seen her in years.

Lying a few feet from this man, I overheard his life story, and it made me sadder and sadder as it unspooled. He had enjoyed a successful career in the tech industry and was able to buy his own condo and retire early. But he never had a family and one by one the people he worked with and hung out with after hours dropped out of his life. Until he was so alone that he had even lost the will to leave his apartment and buy food for himself. I had never heard such a lonesome story in my life.

My family has a history of taking in strays and outcasts, but I was in no position to expand its loving circle. At that point, I was more dead than alive. And my family was beset with woes rippling from my calamity. In any case, my hospital roommate was gone the next day. I still wonder what became of him.

Despite my feeble, disoriented state, the two days and nights on the hellish third floor quickly indoctrinated in me an understanding of the hospital as a workplace filled with anguish, macabre humor and humdrum routine. Modern hospitals are Lysol-washed factories. They have round-the-clock eight-hour shifts and work rules and protocols and labor grievances and human grudges and bitchiness. By the time I was mercifully transferred to a cheery, sunny room on the stroke ward, the fog had begun to lift from my embattled brain, and I was getting a sense of the daily grind around me and the personalities of the women and men on whom I was now utterly dependent.

The Davies Campus of California Pacific Medical Center, which occupies a small area tucked away on the edge of the Castro district, has something of a legendary reputation as one of the main treatment centers for the AIDS epidemic that ravaged San Francisco in the 1980s and '90s—a plague that brought out the city's true glory and human solidarity. The stroke ward staff, and the hospital in general, still has glimmers of this brave past.

On the stroke floor, I was quickly swarmed by neurology doctors, nurses, physical therapists and speech specialists. I presented something of a challenge to the stroke team, as I lay sprawled semi-conscious in bed, seeing double and unable to stand on my own, my speech twisted and labored, my throat muscles stricken and unable to swallow even liquids without great difficulty, and my right-side limbs half-paralyzed and as heavy as barbells. But my energetic rehab team had me working my damaged mind and body as soon as I moved to the stroke floor, as if they were preparing me to compete in the Paralympic Games.

My strenuous daily regimen was printed out the night before and taped to my bedside wall. A shower in the morning, followed by breakfast—each of which normally pleasant introductions to the day required strenuous effort and discipline. Then there was a relentless lineup of time slots devoted to walking, with the help of a leg brace, rolling walker and even a ceiling pulley; step-climbing and other exercises in the gym; arranging blocks and solving puzzles in the game room, to reestablish the neural connection between my brain and limbs; wordplay meant to improve my garbled speech, with some sounds like those beginning with "s" proving especially elusive; and equally frustrating efforts to write, using a right hand that felt more like a claw. This exhausting rehab routine was punctuated by rounds of pharmaceutical infusions through a feeding tube, injections in my stomach, and blood tests when suitable veins could be found in my arms or hands.

I worked this daily regimen as hard as I could, only rarely pleading the fatigue that I chronically felt, because I knew that a stroke patient's wounded brain is particularly responsive to healing stimulus in the first weeks of recovery. But I also sweated and strained because most members of the stroke team were so inspiring and I didn't want to let them down. They seemed so young and good-looking and vibrant that to disappoint them would have meant giving up on life itself. They were my new family members. I grew so quickly attached to them that it felt like I'd known them for years.

The deliriously diverse makeup of the stroke ward staff was the most powerful answer imaginable to the cramped, walled world of Trump-style nationalism. The doctors and nurses and technicians and therapists come from all around the world: Guatemala, Brazil, China, the Philippines, Ethiopia, Russia, Germany, Tasmania and beyond. They were lesbian, gay, straight and none of the above. And they all treated me as a human being worth their time and care.

Humor became our daily bond and salve. I soon realized how grim their work could be and how they needed to laugh as much as I did. During cracks in our relentless routines, one or two of the stroke ward team members would sit on my bed and tell me scandalous jokes. They gossiped about their hospital unit and the holiday parties that were being planned, and asked my advice about whether they should stay with friends in Palm Springs for Christmas, even though they had mixed feelings about the guest list. They shared outrageous stories about hospital life—like the patient who was equipped with a bowel bag but couldn't help eating a smuggled-in bean burrito, with explosive consequences. It took the hazmat team days to clean his room.

The stroke team expanded my traditional Western medical treatment, with all its latest pharmacology and intrusive devices, by offering me an array of alternative care, from acupuncture to Reiki. Even though I had avoided all unconventional types of healing in the past, I quickly agreed to sample every treatment method offered me, no matter how esoteric. Who knew what would help me? One especially creative male nurse named Glenn took to adorning the center of my body with gemstones. (It felt warm and comforting.) A neurosurgeon who happened to come into my room during one such treatment was stunned by the tableau that greeted him—it looked like I was being prepared for human sacrifice.

Among my numerous disabilities after my stroke was urinary dysfunction. My inability to piss forced the nurses to catheterize me three or four times a day. This procedure is, of course, not something to look forward to, and as the dread time would draw near, I would dearly pray that I would get one of the more adept nurses on duty. The gay nurses tended to be best at wielding a catheter. "Honey, I know my way around a penis," one of my favorite nurses assured me. "The trick is to use lots of lube. You're going to be so lubed up you'll hardly feel a thing." Which turned out to be sort of true. Sort of.

As the days and weeks wore on, despite the nurses' ungrudging assistance, I began to worry more and more about my equipment failure. My worst fear was that when I was finally discharged from the hospital, I still wouldn't be able to, well, discharge. As the date drew near, in fact, the nursing staff began to prepare me for this unhappy possibility by trying to train my wife and me to do the procedure. But I proved inept because my right arm and hand were still benumbed. Poor Camille seemed grimly game to learn the task.

I'm delighted to announce (you can't imagine how delighted) that just days before I was due to be released, the floodgates opened and the golden fluid flowed. When at long last I pissed on my own, the nursing staff—who had the sweet but sort of annoying habit of asking me how it went each time I visited the bathroom—broke into loud cheers in my room. For the rest of the day, doctors and nurses filed into my room to congratulate me. The blessed event occurred ten days before Christmas, and it was the best present I've ever had. Truly.

The holiday season was made much more festive for me when I was visited by my sister Margaret, who had flown in from the East Coast, where she writes for the *New Yorker* magazine. One evening Margaret and Camille brought some sparkling Christmas lights to decorate my hospital room. I had requested lavender lights instead of the traditional red and green (boring). Eliano, my male nurse from Brazil, was a larger-than-life, boisterous presence, and he insisted on re-stringing the lights and rearranging the get-well bouquets that kept arriving, in order to make the room more fabulous. He succeeded beyond my wildest dreams. Later, when I was getting ready to leave, he demanded that I gift the lavender lights to him, and I couldn't imagine a better home for them.

Confined to the stroke ward day after day, week after week, it was crucial for me to transform my functional-looking room during the evenings by bathing it in a warm, theatrical glow and by playing the music mixes my family brought me. The redesign was my way of making myself feel more at home—and more like myself instead of a medical victim. My room also became an oasis for the worn-out stroke ward staff, who seemed cheered up by the twinkling lights and soft music when they stopped by on their rounds.

The deep, dark hours of the night are naturally the most disturbing in a hospital. The hustle and bustle has died out, and all you hear is the occasional eerie moan from another patient's room, some suffering soul who can't make it through the night. It's hard to slumber in peace because you're awakened at regular intervals by nurses who need to "check your vitals," to make sure you're still alive. The graveyard shift at hospitals is sometimes staffed by heroic individuals—and at times by some of the sketchier personnel, those who seem too old, or frankly odd, to be doing this kind of strenuous, late-hour labor.

About halfway through my hospitalization, I was very fortunate to have a true shining angel appear by my bedside during the after-midnight shift. She often had the unenviable task of catheterizing me in the wee wee hours, which she invariably did with expert hands and remarkably good cheer. During odd intervals like this, I often fell into conversation with the nurses, asking about their background stories—out of journalistic habit, loneliness and a genuine curiosity to know about the men and women who held my life, and my body parts, in their hands. This particular angel, whom I never saw in a bad mood during my long weeks in the hospital, had come to San Francisco from the Philippines as a young woman. Now she was a grandmother, and she regaled me with stories about her family and about the holiday feasts she was planning. One night she brought me her homemade tapioca pudding because she knew I had a hard time swallowing.

Eventually it came out that this woman cared for her autistic grandson during her off hours from the hospital. While encouraging me to learn how to catheter myself, she told me that her brother had been crippled in a car accident as a young man, and had been forced to learn to catheter himself many years ago because he was paralyzed from the waist down. She told me that her buoyant spirit came from her Catholic faith, but there was something holier even deeper in her soul.

It's funny—I can't remember her name now, which seems fitting in a way. This nurse's visitations in the ghostly hours of the night still fill me with dreamlike memories.

I could go on forever about my hospital family. About Nella, the young, strong and beautiful Cambodian-American physical therapist whose parents had escaped the mad killing fields there. Nearly a foot shorter than I am, Nella forced me to stand when I thought my swirling dizziness would make me throw up. And she had me walking with a cane when I thought I'd never take another step, catching me in a flash with her sturdy arm whenever I started to tip over.

And there was Rebecca, my speech therapist, the progeny of a Jewish father and Chinese-American mother who had met in the trenches of City Hall politics (classic San Francisco story). Rebecca began each morning by reading to me from the daily newspapers, because she knew I was a news junkie. She encouraged me to eat increasingly more challenging solid foods, carefully watching my throat muscles with each swallow to make sure I didn't choke or aspirate. At this stage of my recovery, eating just a few morsels was so arduous, and frankly scary, that it hardly seemed worth it. Rebecca was another miracle worker on the stroke patient "reassembly line"—a young woman so boundless in her radiance and determination that it was infectious. At a time when my facial paralysis made it nearly impossible to even crack a crooked smile, she made me laugh out loud about the latest Trump antics or some other absurdity of life.

During my long residence in the Davies hospital stroke ward, I began to rebuild myself, slowly and painstakingly. While there, I realized I would never be the same as I was before, that I had changed forever. But I also learned I was still a recognizable version of myself, and in some ways a better version. The stroke ward staff not only restored my faith in myself and my ability to keep healing, but in the future itself. At a time when everything seems broken, most of all the American health-care system, this rainbow team of men and women from all over the world worked in remarkable harmony, performing large and small acts of grace and kindness on a daily basis. They not only made it possible for me to keep living; they restored my faith in the often questionable phenomenon that is the human race.

CHAPTER 5

A CHRISTMAS MIRACLE

While I was floating in the weird but comforting womb of the Davies stroke ward, the outside world rarely intruded. My daily worries were generally of a mundane nature—like when could I start drinking liquids without a nauseating, gelatinous thickener added to each drink so that I could swallow without choking. (Strangely, though I was chewing more challenging foods as the weeks went by, liquids that rushed too quickly down my gullet were still a big worry.) But as my release date, scheduled for shortly before Christmas, drew near, my outside world anxieties again began assailing me.

Money worries have plagued me through most of my life as a freelance writer and media entrepreneur. I learned to handle this chronic economic uncertainty at an early age, as the son of an actor. Perhaps "handle" is too glib a word—"weather" this constant upheaval is more accurate.

My father, Lyle Talbot, began performing during his teens as a magician's apprentice in the early part of the twentieth century and then as the young leading man in a theater troupe that traveled throughout the American heartland. In 1932, he was on stage in Dallas when a Warner Brothers talent scout discovered him, leading to a fairy-tale movie career as a lover and gangster (or both), co-starring with the likes of Humphrey Bogart, Bette Davis, Barbara Stanwyck and Spencer Tracy during Hollywood's Golden Age. After a postwar dive into booze and middle-age doldrums, he was revived by his much younger, vivacious wife Paula (my mother), and began a second career as the genial neighbor and sidekick on the TV sitcoms of my youth like *The Adventures of Ozzie and Harriet*.

My dad always had a saying when things looked low: "Something will turn up." It was a blind optimism born of his plucky Irish heritage and his usual show business good fortune. But when days or weeks went by with no phone calls from his agent, his confidence would begin to erode and a chill crept over the house.

Years later, as I struggled to pursue my own career dreams and to provide for my family, I weathered the same ups and downs my father had. I learned to ride the emotional waves, but over time all the cresting and crashing had taken its toll on me and my family. We realized this is what it took to lead a creative life, to be a member of the "Talbot Players," as my father named his touring theater troupe decades before. But all of us—including Camille and our two sons—sometimes wondered if this exciting, free life was worth all the tension.

I tried not to worry about money when I was in the hospital. After all, it was chronic stress that had helped put me there. But the old anxiety loomed larger as I surfaced from the underwater depths of my stroke. I knew I couldn't return anytime soon, or maybe ever, to writing the ambitious history book I was under contract to finish in a year. I still couldn't even type. And Camille knew she now had to help care for me, taking a long leave from her own book-in-progress, the romantic and literary odyssey of Fanny and Robert Louis Stevenson. *Something will turn up, something will turn up*, I kept whispering to myself late at night in my hospital bed. But with the revenue pipeline suddenly turned off for both Camille and me, it was hard to see from where this fortune would flow.

Then, in a burst of family inspiration, something did turn up. The idea would not have occurred to me, but my son Joe was more generationally in tune with the crowd-funding concept. Working with my sister Margaret, Joe wrote a heartfelt plea for donations, sharing the news of my medical trauma and our family's financial plight. Our dear family friend Ruth Henrich posted the appeal on a GoFundMe web page. It was a message in a bottle tossed into the waves, a desperate and even embarrassing gambit, to me at least. But my family *was* desperate. Fortunately my head still felt too groggy for me to worry about my reputation or the response that the soul-baring open letter would elicit.

To my everlasting gratitude, the responses from family, friends and complete strangers who knew me only through my writing and political activism immediately began coming in, at first in a trickle and then in a gush. I could read only with great difficulty at this point, with printed words gliding before my eyes like gray wisps of clouds. So at the end of each day, Camille or

Joe would read to me the messages that were flowing in to the GoFundMe page along with donations. They made me laugh or cry, or both at the same time. My emotions were as volatile as a summer mountain storm. The flood of mail reminded me of past glories and fiascos in my life, of loves lost and forever won. Hearing my life memorialized in these messages made me feel like Tom Sawyer, hiding in the church gallery and eavesdropping on his own funeral.

My family raised over $40,000 from dozens of contributors during the GoFundMe drive. The money made a crucial difference, bridging us to the date, months in the future, when my state disability payments finally began arriving, and then helping cover our living expenses when those disability checks proved insufficient. But it's the personal notes that accompanied these donations, some of which were mailed to the hospital or left on my family's doorstep, that I'll always remember.

One of my favorite handwritten notes that arrived at the hospital came from a former *Salon* colleague with whom I hadn't been in touch since he left for a more majestic publication many years ago. I was never fully certain how to act as a boss when I launched *Salon*. Most of the *Salon* staff was made up of friends and drinking mates, or friends of these friends. But this letter assured me that I ran a good ship, that I was "so upbeat and funny and good-weird." He concluded his note by writing, "You also smelled so damn good, too"—a strange but lovely encomium that I want chiseled on my tombstone. I was especially delighted to read of my pleasing aroma while confined to the stroke ward, where showers were an every-two-or-three-day treat.

I was also deeply moved by a graceful little handwritten card attached to a bouquet of flowers that arrived for Camille, whose emotional blows seemed unending at the time. While I was hospitalized, she was shuttling back and forth between my stroke ward and a nursing home near Sacramento where her ninety-four-year-old mother, Alice, was slowly dying. Alice took her last breath late one night as Camille and her brother Don sat by her bedside. After Alice's death, the tiny card that arrived for Camille read simply: "For Camille: A small sentiment from someone who has yet to meet you. Your strength & grace is felt miles away. Thinking of you and your family every day."

How can you read a mysterious note like this and *not* believe in humanity—in people's bewildering and beautiful capacity to comfort and uplift?

That's why I say that in some wondrous way my stroke beatified my life. My head cracked open one evening in November 2017; but I have been filled with an ineffable light and joy ever since. All around me, America was rife with anger and rancor; you couldn't help choking on the acrid air. But when I was broken and my family was helpless, we were swept up by angels, known and unknown, who carried us gracefully aloft.

CHAPTER 6

A CHRISTMAS MIRACLE 2

My house felt like an Airbnb rental to me when I came home on the afternoon of December 22. I'd been so far away in the past five weeks, further than just the hospital; I was submerged in such an eerie shadow world that I felt like a visitor in my own home of twenty-five years.

I was overcome with this sense of alienation despite everything my family had done to welcome me home. While caring for me at the hospital, my wife and sons had gone to the seasonal trouble of buying and trimming a Christmas tree and decorating our house with holiday cheer. And my family had worked hard to make our house not only Christmas cozy, but also navigable for me by installing safety rails along the front doorsteps and in the bathroom, and by equipping me with a wheelchair, walker, cane and safety socks that gripped the floor.

Camille, Joe and Nat doted on me, and so did our circle of love. A close friend brought trays of steaming lasagna from a favorite old-fashioned Italian restaurant in San Francisco's Sunset district; other friends and neighbors delivered home-made casseroles, soups and ribbon-wrapped tins filled with fresh-baked Christmas cookies and chocolates.

All this human warmth was essential; it began to thaw the chill of death inside me. But I must be honest about this transitional period of my life. It wasn't until our dog, Brando, worked up the courage to jump on my bed and welcome me that I felt truly at home. I was sleeping downstairs, in my son Joe's bedroom, because I still couldn't easily climb the stairs to Camille's and my bedroom. This was one of the strange new arrangements that Brando had to figure out. Weirder still, I had suddenly reappeared in our house after an inexplicably long absence.

Brando had been able to see me once in the hospital, on a special dog-visiting Sunday. His cameo appearance on the stroke ward was very popular with staff and patients. Brando, who lives up to his name, has a certain star appeal. A mix between a Labrador, a standard poodle, and God knows what else, he looks like "the kind of dog that Disney would order from central casting," as one fellow dog walker once observed. Brando has floppy, velvety ears and a thick, rusty-red coat with adorable white markings, including a stripe down the middle of his regal snout, spats on all four paws and a snowy ascot on his chest. His eyes, and eyebrows, seem particularly alert and expressive. And no, it's not just me who thinks he expertly uses them to communicate his wide range of emotions.

Brando's a very empathetic animal, and my wife and I call petting his plush coat "fur therapy." When family members argue loudly or shout at the TV during a frustrating ball game, Brando inevitably lays a heavy, therapeutic paw on the angry person's lap, as if telling him or her to calm down, all this heated temper is not healthy. And he doesn't remove the paw until the person actually starts relaxing. So, naturally, Camille thought a hospital visit would be good for both of us.

But the strange environment—with its whooshing elevators and scary, rumbling machines—discombobulated Brando. He came slipping and sliding into my room on the slick hospital floors, and he didn't quite know what to make of me. I must have smelled of medication and distress to him. He seemed relieved to get the hell out of there after his brief visit.

But weeks later, at home, despite my still-drooping face and weird glasses, Brando could sense that some Christmas miracle had happened. I was gone, maybe forever—then I was suddenly home. It seemed like he couldn't let himself believe it. Nor could I. At first he didn't know what to make of my mysterious reappearance. Then, as I settled down to sleep in my borrowed bed that first night home, Brando did something he had never done before. He jumped onto the bed, burrowed under the covers with me, and put his paw on my shoulder while looking directly into my wounded eyes. "I can't believe it's you—I can't believe you've really come home," he seemed to be saying.

He slept every night on my bed for the next two months, to make sure I wasn't going anywhere.

During the daytime, when I began my walking exercises, Brando continued his vigil. As I lurched from one end of the house to the other—at first with the aid of a walker on tennis balls and later with a cane—Brando would dutifully pad right behind me, even if another human was overseeing me, as if to make sure I could stay upright.

In the days and weeks after I arrived home, Brando and I grew closer than ever because we spent so much time together and it seemed like we now had a similar status in life. My disabled existence has given me enormous new sympathy for Brando. I've become acutely aware of how dependent he is on others for a wide spectrum of basic needs, like eating, drinking and when and where to relieve himself. Not to mention transportation to and from the pet doctor, and a whole range of daily amusements, like trips to the park and beach, and fun rides in the car. I identify more with Brando these days, and the frustrating limitations in his life, because of my own new circumscribed conditions.

Through our deeper bonding, I've developed a more neural feeling for Brando's own distress. As he's grown older, he's become increasingly frightened by loud explosions, particularly barrages of fireworks. Unfortunately San Franciscans leap at any excuse to light up the sky, not waiting for Fourth of July but launching legal and illegal rockets on New Year's Eve, Chinese New Year, Cinco de Mayo and other holidays, and at various ballpark celebrations and music festivals. Brando starts shivering and panting heavily at the opening salvo of these booming celebrations, as the adrenaline rushes through his body. In his terror, he has begun jumping on my bed and laying his head and front paws across my chest for comfort. It's as if he needs to feel the beating of my heart to regain his own rhythm. He makes me feel, despite all my physical loss, that I'm still an alpha dog and can still protect him from the shock and awe of life.

CHAPTER 7

THE MEDITATIONS
OF MR. TOAD

A fter I returned home and slowly grew stronger—less dizzy and nauseated—I felt an increasing urge to reengage with life. But I quickly learned that I had to regulate this reentry for the good of my health. The slow pace of my revival was frustrating at times, but my body could only be pushed so far—and it quickly alerted me to its limits via my blood pressure readings, which I was taking each morning on my portable electronic Omron machine.

I tend to run hot, or at least I used to. My body literally gave off waves of heat—or so I've been told by those who've had the comfort of my body in their beds on cold nights. Similarly, when I throw myself into journalism or politics, I'm known to get a bit . . . heated. The stakes of engagement always seem so high to me; so much human anguish—or salvation—hangs in the balance in this constant clash of ideas.

Strokes, however, have a tendency to reset your life—or at least give you the opportunity to do so. While I was a patient on the stroke ward, my physical therapists were always instructing me to move slower. I had a tendency to lunge instead of slowly rising from bed to a standing position. They would call my sudden upward movements "launching." *Whoa, whoa, whoa, big guy*, they were constantly reminding me, *slow your roll*.

I've long been fond of the children's classic *The Wind in the Willows*. At the hospital, Camille, my brother, Steve, and sister-in-law, Pippa, would come read to me from a dog-eared paperback copy of the book. My brother, an award-winning public TV producer who was a child actor, read his lines with theatrical zest. And Pippa, a home-care social worker of British–South African heritage, read with a properly plummy accent. In my medical duress, these bedside readings— conjuring up a more halcyon world of wild English meadows and amusing river creatures—were deeply comforting to me. The book oddly took me back to childhood, though I hadn't discovered the timeless tale until I was grown up. In any case, early in our marriage, Camille pegged me as a Mr. J. Thaddeus Toad, the book's irrepressible main character, forever being swept up in splendid manias and trying to drag his long-suffering mates along with him. Toad is always crying out, "Come! I'll show you the world!"

This kind of manic behavior has energized my life and has given me the pluck (or madness) to do ambitious things . . . like starting *Salon*, at a time when most people still thought the World Wide Web was some sort of international tennis tournament. Or trying to solve the JFK assassination, by following his brother Bobby's secret investigative path and plumbing the deep fractures between the Kennedy administration and its national security state. An epic American tragedy.

I'm proud of these grand ventures, but they took a toll on me. As I wrote earlier, we were forever fighting to keep *Salon* alive, under constant financial and political pressures. And challenging the massively constructed official story of the Kennedy assassination demanded a similar zealous spirit, including a willingness to blow up my bridges to safer media and political shores.

That's where the Mr. Toad in me came in handy. He urged me to plunge forward when caution bid me to hesitate or stop.

After years of combat in the public arena, it was hard for me to slow down. When I was in the hospital, Rebecca, my speech therapist, was always urging me to be less Toad, and more tortoise. She drew a tortoise on the wall-length mirror in my hospital bedroom, where nurses wrote the names of my family members and their phone numbers, along with the day of the week and date, in case my scrambled brain couldn't recall the information.

I've found—late in life—that meditating in the morning before I get out of bed helps turn down my body's thermostat. Hitting the ground running now sounds to me like a recipe for a bad day. I have absolutely no background in meditation, but I love how my stroke has derailed my life in surprising ways.

I embarked on my new meditation regimen by adopting an exercise ritual after waking each morning. If I skip the exercises, which I do while still flat on my back in bed, I'm more wobbly on my feet and my heart tends to race as I begin my day.

I hold one knee in an upright position for thirty seconds with clasped hands, then bend it toward my navel for another half minute, before repeating the routine with my other knee. This helps eliminate the chronic lower back pain that was becoming worse before I learned this exercise in a post-stroke physical therapy class. I also perform an exercise I learned in the hospital that strengthens my core—lifting my pelvis in the air without using my arms for support and feeling my stomach muscles tighten. While I practice my exercises, I avoid frantically plotting the new day as I would have in the past; instead I sleepily recall moments of pleasure from my previous day. I suppose I'm savoring time these days, so what's left of my life doesn't rush away from me.

One day, I suddenly felt compelled to go searching on Amazon for *Ram Dass, Fierce Grace*, the 2001 documentary that spiritual teacher Ram Dass made about his stroke. Ram Dass, of course, was Richard Alpert in a former life and was fired back in 1963 from Harvard's psychology department, along with Timothy Leary, for conducting psychedelic drug experiments. Although I was only passingly familiar with Ram Dass's life story and spiritual journey, I was inclined to learn from him. As he explains in *Fierce Grace*, he was born about fifteen years before baby boomers like me started arriving on earth, so he has long acted as a spiritual tour guide for my generation. After suffering his stroke at age sixty-six, Ram Dass was given the opportunity to share his wisdom about this mind-blowing trip too, since he knew that many of us younger ones would be following in his broken path soon enough.

One of Ram Dass's drops of insight that struck me just right was his admonition not to try living your life the same way as before your stroke. Trying to return to your former life will only bring frustration and despair, he cautioned. It's true. I now feel deeply different, like my head is inside a bell jar. And so I have to live differently, more softly, or that bell jar will shatter.

In *Still Here*, the memoir about his stroke that inspired the documentary, Ram Dass writes of eventually achieving a higher consciousness as a result of his stroke, less caught up in the "Ego world" of ambition, desire and fear, and more attuned to the deeper humming of his "Soul world," where he makes peace with his new physical reality and lets his mind wander to higher places.

"I'm taking more risk with my consciousness these days," Ram Dass writes. "I can let the kite-string out a lot farther. It's scary sometimes, it's like going into outer space, and you're afraid of getting lost out there. Sometimes I'll find my consciousness someplace and I'll ask myself, 'Now how did I get here?' I let myself get farther away from home plate than ever."

As I've slowly felt my way into my new life, I've begun looking into meditation classes at the San Francisco Zen Center. And, in my amateurish way, I created a mantra that helps calm me as I meditate in the morning, during my bed exercises. The mantra popped into my head as I prepared to take an overnight trip to Point Reyes, the national park hugging the Pacific coastline north of San Francisco, one of my happiest places on earth. It was my first visit to Point Reyes since my "rather unfortunate incident," as I sometimes refer to my medical trauma, Blanche DuBois style. I was thinking of Point Reyes's beautiful collage of forest, meadows and sea when the mantra found its way into my brain:

"Be the water, be the trees, be the sunshine, be the breeze."

83

Repeating this slowly, over and over, settles my overly active brain as I fully wake each morning.

I'm a thoroughly urban person, but there's something mystical about Point Reyes that utterly transports my Celtic soul. It's where I want my ashes to be scattered after I die, into the wind over Tomales Bay. (*"Be the water . . ."*)

Soon after I returned home from the hospital, friends sent me a very moving essay about Walt Whitman, who suffered a stroke in his fifties and lived nearly twenty more years. Whitman extended his life by giving up his day job as a government paper-pusher in Washington, D.C., and settling into a very active retirement in Camden, New Jersey, and the surrounding countryside. Nature, he wrote, was a balm to his wounded mind and his soul.

Of course I can't give up all journalism and politics—all the friction in my life. It's a life force that keeps me going; it's who I am. But I've come to understand that what I love is also what's killing me. And so certain adjustments need to be made—I have to learn how to engage with life, but in a more restrained way. "Life flows on within you and without you"—George Harrison understood this essential dichotomy. We are burning with life, but our lives are small and finite in the face of the infinite. Feeling this eternal contradiction deep inside helps me live my life with more balance and perspective.

The fact is, I'm physically and psychologically incapable of pursuing life the way I once did. For one thing, I have to eat more slowly in order not to choke—which of course helps me savor my meals. Room temperature water, sluicing too quickly down my throat, sends me into coughing fits. And when I walk into a restaurant, movie theater lobby or political meeting—anywhere in public—I always feel that my entire presence screams "invalid." I walk with a cane and my vision is still broken and disturbed.

Because of the swirling weirdness in my head, I just don't feel like my old self—and the feeling is growing within me that I never will. I'm a strange half-and-half creature. Life goes on within me and without me.

I can tell that this twilight existence of mine freaks out some of my old friends. "I just hate to see you this way!" blurted out one old acquaintance on seeing me recently—he remembers me plowing through life with a lot more vigor. It sounded oddly insensitive to me at the time, but it made me smile one of my stroke-induced crooked smiles. I know what he meant—it takes some adjustment to be with me, not just to be me.

I now live in a ghost world, and not everyone who was once close to me wants to venture into this shadowy place to hang out with me. Some people are clearly spooked. I remind them of their own frailty and mortality. I get it; it's understandable. But it confirms my spectral status to me.

———

Even stranger are the friends who act as if nothing has changed, like I'm still the same old David Talbot. I sort of am, but I'm not. Trying to act like my old self takes a lot out of me, and in the end it's not worth it. After these visits, I feel drained and lost to myself.

I enjoy the company of family and friends who can engage in bursts of banter with me, like in the old days, and then can just sit by my side and let things drift quietly for a while. And who drop ice cubes in my glass of water, because they know that room-temperature drinks can make me choke. The truth is, I want to keep living at half-speed, in my secure, bubble world, with those to whom I can feel effortlessly close. No, I don't just want to—I *need* to.

I feel more spirit than flesh these days. So here's another mantra that I've begun whispering to myself: *"All the frenzy, all the woe, embrace life, let it go."* It helps me come to terms with the fragile new me. It helps me keep going.

CHAPTER 8

DANCE THERAPY

My stroke has made me clumsy. I feel like I'm staggering instead of walking sometimes, particularly when I'm tired. I have depth perception problems. I bump into things, and knock over objects with arms and hands that feel slightly out of control, like they have a faulty guidance system. The other day, while eating lunch, I jabbed my fork into the inside of my cheek, which produced a singularly unpleasant sensation I'd never felt before. Going shopping, or undertaking any public outing in a crowded place, is always an adventure, carrying with it equal amounts of risk and weirdly giddy fun.

During a recent visit to the market, I picked up a big plastic jar of store-made chicken soup for an ailing friend, only to feel the slick container slip inexorably through my grasp and plummet to the floor in a geyser of chicken chunks, carrots and broth. Oops. Clean-up on Aisle Four.

Some of this physical awkwardness is due to my "vision deficit," as my therapists call it. My stroke resulted in pontine gaze palsy, meaning my left eye is out of orbit, with the pupil drifting toward my nose, like a satellite gone haywire. My right eye, thankfully, remains largely normal—although I've needed reading glasses for many years. I'm now waiting for new prescription glasses that I hope will greatly help my vision. But the truth is, though I've come a long way with the help of my rehab therapists, I don't expect to come fully back. For bad, and good, I'm not the person I once was.

So given this physical toll on me, it came as something of a rebirth to find that I'm suddenly a dancing fool. About once a day, my damaged body breaks into joyous, somewhat unhinged, movement.

In fact, I'm dancing more these days than I have since the 1980s, when I was a regular on the San Francisco dance club circuit. Those were wild and free nights, before my wife and I started making a family. Clubs like the I-Beam and the Stud and DNA Lounge and Paradise Lounge and the Oasis were our playground. The AIDS epidemic was beginning to stalk the party, like the specter of Red Death at Edgar Allan Poe's masquerade ball. But the city's nightlife was still filled with revelry in gay and straight and mixed dance clubs.

Maybe I break into dance these days for the same reason we did back then. Because I'm still alive and that feeling throbs inside me every day. Because it's a fuck-you to illness and infirmity and death.

Recently Camille and my sister Margaret took me shopping at Unionmade, a men's clothes store in the Castro district where the apparel is "responsibly manufactured" but as a result is very pricey. It wasn't exactly a shopping spree—we can't afford that—but I bought a couple of T-shirts and a short-sleeve shirt for the coming warm weather. While I was there, trying on clothes in the dressing room with my two gal pals, the store soundtrack suddenly erupted with dance tunes from the '80s. Bronski Beat! Boy George! Yaz! Soft Cell! Echo and the Bunnymen!

Without any warning, my awkward, vision-impaired body turned into Party Boy, a.k.a. Strokey, one of my new alter egos. I was seized by the irresistible music and started dancing in the dressing area like it was 1984. Camille and Margaret were initially taken aback, but Party Boy's infectious joy is hard to resist. Soon the three of us had turned the store into our own private Idaho.

Safety tip: I must interject that stroke survivors should endeavor to dance close to loved ones—or next to a sofa or bed, as I do when dancing at home—in case your dance mania sends you sprawling. I have to confess that I tend to dance with what former Federal Reserve Chairman Alan Greenspan once called "irrational exuberance." By the way, he wasn't referring to my dancing, but to the stock market.

My stroke has transported me back to a more fun and more physical me, in part by stripping a significant amount of weight from my body. In the beginning, the pounds just melted away—hospital food and medication overloads and chronic nausea will combine to do that. Now the pounds are disappearing more slowly, but they still are gradually melting, as food has taken on a different meaning in my life. I cook at home more often now, and I carefully plan each meal, as something to savor and to delight my family, rather than to simply recharge my stressed-out body.

Also, I'm not supposed to drink alcohol because my head and body are already in tipsy mode, so I don't get any calories in liquor form. That too has been a surprisingly easy transition. I don't miss the martinis that fueled a lot of my journalism life, but at some point I can see easing a good glass of wine back into my dinner routine. On some warm evenings a favorite rosé calls out to me, or a crisp Chablis.

I gained weight slowly and surely over the years after I got married, while raising children with my wife, and girding for battle in the worlds of online journalism and partisan politics. I think my extra weight was body armor against the daily storm that seemed to increase as my career picked up steam, and America became more discordant, and my family grew—and along with it the financial pressures.

Now that my body is lighter, however, I'm lighter in spirit too—both of which make it easier for me to break into dance. As I've observed before, my stroke has made me feel that I'm no longer fully in this world. Much of my existence is spent in some strange twilight zone. I feel like Jon Snow in *Game of Thrones*—brought back to life from death through some dark magic, but bewildered and unsettled by this resurrection. I'm still searching for the meaning in my stroke of fortune, when it was probably just dumb luck that I was revived.

Dancing serves a dual, and contradictory, purpose in my new life. On the one hand, it roots me to this life, makes me feel its sensual pulse. For some reason, following my brain attack, I could suddenly hear the drumbeat in songs much more clearly and strongly. I could tell when the beat was slightly off or too loud, even though I have no background in drumming at all. Paging Dr. Sacks!

Speaking of Oliver Sacks, while dancing grounds me in this world, it can also make me higher and put me in touch with another world. A more celestial place—where the late literary neurologist hopefully now resides. The good doctor was taught the endless wonders of disrupted brains such as mine by his fascinating patients.

If there is any meaning to my resurrection, I feel that it's to bring more joy into the lives of those I love and care about. That's where Party Boy comes in. He's always ready to, well, party—even when his limbs are out of control. And giving in to dance fever at weird and inopportune times, particularly in public, has a way of making loved ones kind of cringe at first in embarrassment, but then give in to the sheer madness of life. Because if your brain can be hit by a bolt of lightning out of the blue, life is completely tenuous and serendipitous. So you might as well dance your ass off.

Postscript: During my dance spree in Broken Brain Land, I've begun to archive the best dance tunes on my laptop. I like to say that these beat-heavy songs are not for stroke survivors, but for stroke *thrivers*. See the Appendix for my dance list, which I call "Songs for Strokeys."

CHAPTER 9

THOMAS MERTON AND THE LIGHT WITHIN

D ivers know that they can't swim to the surface too quickly or they might suffer the bends. As I've written, I soon realized that if I propelled myself upward too aggressively from my post-stroke depths, my head—which sometimes feels as fragile as an eggshell—could crack again from the pressure. So I need to find the right pace at which to reenter the human race—and the roiling public arenas where I've spent much of my life.

As I recover at home, the outside world is raging so madly that the bedlam can't be blocked out—screaming headlines by the day, by the hour. The national psychodrama feels more urgent and demanding than at any other time in my life, at least since the Vietnam War and Nixon's hovering police state shadowed my youth. But back then, I could run in the streets, I could dodge police clubs and tear gas canisters. Now I must move much slower.

So I made my reentry into the world of street "actions" by joining the 2018 San Francisco demonstration against Trump's family-busting immigration policies, marching at my own speed with the help of the cane that I've anointed "Citizen Kane" or "Raising Cain" in honor of my walking stick's public service. It helped that the protest march's leisurely pace was set by parents pushing baby strollers.

But gauging the right speed of my public resurfacing is more of a mental, even spiritual, exercise than a matter of physical stamina. These days I'm trying to find the right balance between passionate social engagement and quiet contemplation. To do this, I've been seeking out meditation workshops, since quiet reflection does not come easily or naturally for me.

Early one Saturday, Camille drove me to an all-morning meditation training session at the Green Gulch Farm Zen Center in nearby Marin County. I found the first hour or so calming; my anxiety seemed to slowly evaporate as we sat silently in our lotus positions and felt the rising and falling of our breath. My anxieties these days don't usually involve my own professional or physical dilemmas—my stroke seemed to mercifully minimize those old frets and fears. But the turmoil of those I love and care about, and the ambient agony all around me, comes at me in never-ending waves. I seem less able to handle other people's worries because I feel less equipped to help them and protect them in my still fragile state. In fact, I sometimes feel like I'm uselessly on the sidelines of not just human strife, but of my own family's troubles.

In any case, even these collective crises were floating away from me during the first hour of sitting and walking meditation in the Zen Center temple. But this sense of peace didn't last long. After a short break, the group slipped back into the disciplinary straits of another lengthy round of meditation, and I found it harder to calm my restless mind. The rustic building suddenly seemed cold and drafty; my feet felt chilled and my body stiff. Apparently Camille was having an even harder time. Suddenly her face—looking a little frantic—was hovering right before me. "I've got to get out of here," she whispered. She seemed gripped by a sort of panic.

Frankly, I was beginning to feel the same way. After enduring the sort of upheaval that has rocked our family lately, there's only so long you can sit and quietly contemplate the havoc. I wanted to join her as she bolted for the door, but with my impaired eyesight, I wasn't sure I could find the door handle in the temple's gloomy light. An hour or so later, when I joined her on the path that curved through lush Green Gulch Farm all the way down to Muir Beach, with briny gusts of sea air in our faces, we found another type of serenity. You don't always need a spiritual dwelling to find peace.

And you don't always need classes run by Zen masters. Reading the right books at the right times in my life has always provided essential solace and guidance. My search for the proper blend of activism and calm has led me to the life and work of Thomas Merton, the Trappist monk who emerged from twenty-seven years of cloistered life in a monastery in the hills of Kentucky to confront the growing apocalyptic evils of the Cold War. Although he didn't watch TV and newspapers were only a sporadic part of his life, Merton acutely felt the gathering darkness of the outside world by staying in touch through letters with a far-flung network of friends. He realized it was not morally tenable to remain in silent isolation as the world skidded toward nuclear oblivion, so he began sending his painfully sensitive and observant commentaries to small Catholic publications. And when his conservative monastic superiors began censoring these articles, he wrote his thoughts in letters and mailed them to his influential circle of like-minded souls, including Pope John XXIII, Boris Pasternak, Dorothy Day, Ethel Kennedy, Erich Fromm, Walker Percy, Lawrence Ferlinghetti, nuclear physicist Leo Szilard and Shinzo Hamai, the mayor of Hiroshima.

"This country has become frankly a warfare state built on affluence, a power structure in which the interests of big business, the obsessions of the military, and the phobias of political extremists both dominate and dictate our national policy," Merton wrote in January 1963 in a preface to his collected Cold War letters, which he mimeographed and sent to friends. "It also seems that the people of the country are by and large reduced to passivity, confusion, resentment, frustration, thoughtlessness and ignorance, so that they blindly follow any line that is unraveled for them by the mass media."

As Catholic writer and activist James Douglass, author of *JFK and the Unspeakable*, has observed, Merton was so closely attuned to the deeply troubled American psyche—as he fitfully exited and returned to his hermitage within the Abbey of Our Lady of Gethsemani—that he was able to foresee President Kennedy's violent death. JFK, wrote Merton, occupied a position within the sharply divided U.S. power structure that was "sometimes so impossible as to be absurd." Kennedy, he predicted, might "by a miracle" someday "break through" America's military-industrial mass death cult. "But such people are before long marked out for assassination."

As death and tragedy rolled in waves through the 1960s, flooding even his remote monastery, Merton still managed to maintain a sense of inner peace, buoyed by his deep Catholic faith. He knew that he would soon lose his sense of direction in the public arena, as the peace movement and civil rights movement became increasingly radical and infected with American violence, if he didn't listen to the inner voice he had been patiently nurturing for nearly three decades.

"He who attempts to act and do things for others or for the world, without deepening his own self-understanding, freedom, integrity and capacity to love, will not have anything to give others," wrote Merton in an essay later collected in a book titled *Contemplation in a World of Action.* "He will communicate to them nothing but the contagion of his own obsessions, his aggressiveness, his ego-centered ambitions, his delusions about ends and means, his doctrinaire prejudices and ideas. . . . We are living through the greatest crisis in the history of man; and this crisis is centered precisely in the country that has made a fetish out of action and has lost (or perhaps never had) the sense of contemplation. Far from being irrelevant, prayer, meditation and contemplation are of the utmost importance in America today."

And so now, as the Trumpian sound and fury grows louder by the day, along with the agonized cries in reaction, I try to find moments each day during which I calm my frantic mind and withdraw to a quiet place inside me. I couldn't seem to find this oasis of serenity before my stroke, but it became my stroke's gift to me.

In the weeks after my stroke, this feeling of tranquility came automatically to me. My head felt cushioned, like it was tucked inside a carrying case. As a result, the bedlam outside my window was muted. Now I have to consciously draw on this deep peace that came through trauma, to take myself back to my hermitage within.

I'm not religious like Merton, so I don't have his disciplinary aids. But in a way I'm just as devout. I believe in something just as transcendental—in the grand prayer of human liberation. Like salvation, it's a dream that seems forever out of reach, but forever worth the struggle.

Like Merton, I can't imagine life without my belief. It's a belief that demands interludes of deep reflection. It also demands action.

CHAPTER 10

A PERSON, NOT A PATIENT

A fter you're released from the stroke ward, your recovery becomes a different sort of experience—less helpless and more interactive. During my first two months at home, I was still in the remote care of the medical system, visited several times a week by a series of therapists—physical, speech and occupational—who helped me adapt to my new daily life. I attribute my success at staying upright and never falling during my first year of recovery—and not slicing off the tip of a finger with a kitchen knife—to this team of home-visiting therapists, with their briskly dispensed yet warm guidance. (Here's a tip to avoid chopping off your digit while chopping onions: Buy a set of nylon-coated safety knives.)

But even with this constant rotation of home help, my physical improvement was driven primarily by my own intense desire to speak more clearly and to walk more steadily. The domestic therapy team drilled into me how much my recovery depended on my own energetic, disciplined commitment to the process. I sat for hours in front of a mirror, stretching my facial muscles with endless repetitions of sound exercises (*ooh, ooh, ah ah, ee, ee* . . .) and tracing patterns with an ice cube on my slightly sagging left cheek to revive my facial nerves.

While my body slowly grew stronger, I also found myself growing fascinated by the mental process of recovery. I had countless questions about brain injuries and the frontiers of neuroscience, some medical but some verging on the philosophical. My physical therapists could talk with me about some of this cerebral universe. But some of my intellectual hunger required an experienced neurologist—one who knew how to speak with a stroke survivor, not simply as a patient but as a person. I quickly devoured popular literature on the subject, including *My Stroke of Insight*, brain scientist Jill Bolte Taylor's illuminating account of her own stroke, and Ram Dass's *Still Here*, a more spiritual but nonetheless down-to-earth chronicle of his stroke. Both books were filled with little epiphanies and bursts of insight that helped me navigate my way through my hobbled first year.

But my insatiable curiosity about my new condition drove me to want more. I longed for a lengthy conversation with a wise medical counselor, someone gifted with scientific knowledge about the human brain but also in awe of its mysteries. In the hospital, I was lucky enough to have two smart, caring doctors who sat with me and Camille during their rounds on the stroke ward and answered our endless questions. But at that point in my recovery, my most urgent questions were fairly basic—*When the hell will I start pissing without a catheter again?* And *Can my feeding tube be safely removed now?*

Some brain doctors, of course, seem to lack all human empathy—and one of them belonged to my hospital team. One day, this brain surgeon made an abrupt entrance into my hospital room after returning from vacation. He was a big-chested man and he loomed over my bed with such puffed-out physicality that he made me feel even more frail than I was. His manner was clipped and perfunctory, as if he were doing me a grand favor simply by visiting my bedside. After a rote greeting, he began firing a series of questions at me—obviously his standard practice for gauging a patient's post-stroke mental capacity.

What's your name? What day of the week is it? What city are we in? As the hospital staff could've told him, those questions were no problem for me, because of the location and nature of my stroke.

"What's this?" he asked me, fingering one of the weirdly wide lapels on his suit jacket.

"A cheap suit?" I ventured. By now I loathed this man.

"What?" he said.

"Your lapel," I answered. Both of my replies were correct.

The doctor then went on to describe my stroke damage in such stark and cold terms that I was convinced I would be severely and irreparably impaired for the rest of my life. His chilling prognosis left little room for hope. By the time he walked briskly out the door, just minutes after he arrived, I felt like crying.

Fortunately my warm, funny speech therapist, Rebecca, came into my room soon afterward and consoled me. "Did he point to his lapel?" she asked. She knew his bedside routine.

A PERSON, NOT A PATIENT

In truth, the brain can be wondrously adaptable after it survives traumas, even injuries more severe than mine. The brain was once conceived as a hardwired mechanism, and any serious damage to it was assumed to be mechanically disastrous, offering little chance of recovery. But starting in the 1960s and '70s, brilliant researchers began expanding our knowledge of the brain and its ability to creatively rewire itself after suffering injury. "If certain 'parts' failed, then other parts could sometimes take over," writes Dr. Norman Doidge in his book about the frontiers of neuroscience, *The Brain That Changes Itself.* "The machine metaphor, of the brain as an organ with specialized [mechanical] parts, could not fully account for changes the [pioneering] scientists were seeing. They began to call this fundamental brain property 'neuroplasticity,'" notes Doidge.

Recently I came upon some papers from my long stay in the hospital that I had stuffed away in a file drawer. Some of the pages were filled with my signatures and letters from the alphabet that I had scrawled in red marking pen during my hospital physical therapy sessions. In my early PT exercises, the handwriting was childish and barely legible. But as the weeks went by, my handwriting steadily improved until it was quite clear, though stylistically different from my pre-stroke penmanship. The part of my brain that controls hand and wrist dexterity had not suddenly come back to life—those brain cells had been snuffed out forever when the blood clot cut off oxygen to part of my brain stem. But constant handwriting practice helped my brain find new neural pathways to my partially paralyzed right-side extremities.

Fortunately, during my outpatient treatment, I was provided with the medical counselor I sought to help me explore these mental mysteries. One afternoon, Camille and I found ourselves sitting in the office of Dr. Michael Ke at the Davies hospital stroke center. It was the beginning of an ongoing doctor-patient conversation that was illuminating if sometimes bracing. Appointments with Dr. Ke, a neurologist and stroke care specialist, proved to be more educational than medical. The traditional doctor-patient hierarchy quickly dissolved in these sessions as Dr. Ke gently but frankly offered medical insights based on his training and experience and encouraged a lively dialogue.

Camille and I found our appointments with Dr. Ke so helpful that I asked if I could interview him for this book. He graciously agreed, and soon after, we were delving into his life story, including what had drawn him into neurology and stroke care. We began by talking about the brain's remarkable transformative power.

"Some brain tissue might be permanently damaged by a stroke, but the remaining parts are plastic and can develop new circuits that allow functional independence through different mechanisms," Dr. Ke observed. "I was so fascinated by this magnificent hidden life of the brain that I got a PhD in learning and memory, and that led me to go into neurology from a clinical perspective. I made stroke treatment my field because I'm someone who likes to make urgent decisions on the fly— that's emergency situations. I spend 90 percent of my time in the hospital, on emergency cases. The rest of the time I'm here in my office, talking with stroke survivors like you."

———

In his early forties, Dr. Ke is lean and alert, and this afternoon he was wearing his usual down vest over an open-collared shirt,

A PERSON, NOT A PATIENT

seemingly to ward off San Francisco's permanent chill. He projected a feeling of calm intelligence as he patiently answered each question, giving a sense that he had all the time in the world for this conversation despite his frantic schedule.

"The traditional way of viewing the physician-patient interaction is a power dynamic, with the physician holding all the power, information and expertise, and dictating the care plan," he continued. "Patients often walk away from these kinds of medical appointments without understanding the rationale behind the doctor's recommended treatments. I find this pattern of communication disheartening, and at times patronizing, and overall ineffective, particularly at motivating people to be healthy. I consider my role as doctor to be an educator, to help patients understand why I'm making specific recovery recommendations. In the process I hope to establish a relationship, to convey that I care. And in doing so, I'm trying to encourage the patients themselves to care for their own bodies. This is why I think of the healing process as a team effort."

Michael Ke was raised in a Virginia suburb of Washington, D.C., where his father worked as a chemist for the federal government. Both of his parents were immigrants from Taiwan. While he was an undergraduate at the College of William & Mary in Virginia, Ke won a scholarship to study comparative medical disciplines in England, and he was exposed to a range of alternatives to Western medicine, including Chinese and Tibetan practices, Ayurveda, homeopathy and naturopathy.

"One of the most memorable lectures I heard during my scholarship in England was by a physician who argued that the sum of the human brain can't be understood by studying its parts. He said if we took everything we know in science about the brain—the connections and circuits and such—we still would not be able to explain human consciousness. It's a mystery beyond our comprehension."

———————

Even as young Ke continued his medical studies at Stanford University School of Medicine, he was aware of the limitations of formal Western medicine. So when he began practicing medicine, he was determined to blend treatments that "correspond to the Western scientific paradigm with holistic disciplines such as meditation, spirituality, mindfulness and universal balance—alternative techniques that manipulate and change the underlying physical properties of the body.

"In our Davies hospital stroke recovery program, you've actually experienced both these approaches—Western and alternative," Dr. Ke told me. "Recommending a blood thinner, for example, is a Western approach—it's manipulating properties of your blood to prevent clots from forming and causing another stroke. On the other hand, your ongoing physical therapy is a holistic approach. Therapists are working with your emotions and behavior to induce specific patterns of neural activity, which in turn induces 'plasticity,' which is then translated to synaptic changes within your brain. These changes can be long-lasting and hopefully beneficial."

Despite his years of formal medical training and practice, Dr. Ke has a supple enough intellect to still be awed by the secrets of the brain. He seems as eager to learn from his stroke patients' mental and emotional journeys as he is to offer them guidance. He's particularly fascinated by how people in creative professions respond to their life-changing brain attacks.

I was eager to discuss this topic. Recently, browsing the internet, I'd come across artwork created by masterful painters after they had suffered strokes. A surprising number of accomplished artists have endured strokes that have left them paralyzed and even half blind, and yet have managed to find a new approach to the canvas. Among them is one of my favorites, Otto Dix, the great chronicler of Germany's descent into decadence and horror during and after World War I. Dix began painting again—differently but still brilliantly—just four days after suffering a right-side hemispheric stroke that left him severely visually impaired on the left side.

Dr. Ke spoke with great wonder about a stroke patient he treated during his Stanford residency. The man, who was about sixty years old when he suffered his ischemic stroke, was an interior designer. "I was intrigued by this, because the stroke significantly damaged the right hemisphere of his brain, which we think of as the creative hemisphere, the one involved in things like spatial abstraction. I wondered, how is this going to affect his work as a designer? Because, of course, your ability to adapt or not adapt to your new life circumstances after a stroke is such an essential challenge."

After some time in the hospital during his lengthy recovery, the patient grew aware of his mental deficits. But this dawning awareness did not crush his spirit.

"One day I walked into his hospital room and he was redesigning it. His partner was helping him because he still couldn't move very well. The designer was directing how he wanted things hung on the wall to make his room more colorful and attractive, because hospital rooms are . . . well, you know. I wasn't familiar with his design work before his stroke, but from talking with him and his partner it was clear that he still had a strong creative impulse—it was just manifesting itself in different ways. For instance, his partner noticed there was a change in the way he would arrange his utensils and his plates on his eating tray. These small choices are important to someone like an interior designer, and he was still doing these arrangements with precision, just differently."

Of course, some of Dr. Ke's stroke patients can't creatively adapt this way and are frustrated and outraged by their new limitations. These are the patients more prone to bouts of bitterness and depression. Practicing medicine in San Francisco, the hot center of the technology boom, Dr. Ke treats a surprising number of young tech workers.

"I don't know what the exact statistics are related to ten years ago, but in our practice at the stroke center we're seeing a lot of younger folks. It's not simply the stress of their work lives—I think these younger people don't take care of themselves. They're working so hard that they don't eat in healthy ways, they don't exercise, they're overweight. They commonly have high blood pressure and high cholesterol. And often they smoke and use recreational drugs to keep themselves charged. These are people in their thirties and forties—even their twenties—and they have all the stroke risk factors we traditionally see in folks who are seventy. And so . . . they have a stroke. It's becoming more and more common at a shockingly young age."

When younger people do suffer a stroke, their chances of significant physical recovery are greater than they are for older patients. But they often suffer more mental anguish. "It's much more emotionally devastating to have a stroke in the prime age of your life when you can be most productive. These are people who are used to multitasking at rapid speeds. But suddenly a coding task or some other chore that took them an hour to do is now taking six or seven hours. They don't have the ability to operate at the same level they did before, and that obviously affects their mood and spirit. They get anxious and depressed. Some people who were operating at the top level of their companies never seem to adjust and they suffer terribly. If they can't operate the same way as before, they feel their lives are lost. But others do adapt—over time they grow to understand their constraints and the new borders of their lives. And they even flourish in new ways."

I tell Dr. Ke that my own calamity befell me at a strangely opportune time, and that I enjoy my altered new life in some unexpected ways—if "enjoy" is the right word.

"I actually try to educate my patients about that. There is no such thing as 'a good stroke' or a stroke that is 'a blessing.' It's a terrible human trauma. But many of my patients—the ones who aren't severely disabled—come out of it feeling strangely blessed. And I take that opportunity to give them my advice. I tell them, 'You were lucky this time—this was a potentially devastating event, for you and your family. But you were lucky the blood clot ended up in one place and not another, and you didn't die or suffer more brain damage. So you have an opportunity—how are you going to lead the rest of your life?'

"These patients come to my office and sit there with their spouses, who often nod in agreement as I'm giving this little lecture. Their loved ones have been telling them for years, 'Slow down, take better care of yourself.' Of course they didn't listen. But now they've been shaken to their core by the trauma. They realize how frail life is. And they've been given a second chance.

"You know, our strategies for preventing a second stroke are pretty good. We know that if you're on blood pressure medicine, a blood thinner like baby aspirin, a cholesterol medicine if you need it, and you don't smoke—those four things in combination will reduce your stroke risk by 90 percent. Exercising regularly and eating wisely is also a big help.

"So it's up to you. Your life is in your own hands."

CHAPTER 11

SANCTUARY CITY

One December morning after waking up in my room at the Davies hospital stroke ward, I learned that Mayor Ed Lee had suffered a heart attack the previous night while shopping at his local Safeway. He died after being rushed to San Francisco's Mark Zuckerberg General Hospital—named for one of the tech titans he had done so much to court. Once I would have told the nurse who asked my opinion of the mayor exactly what I thought of him. Now I just wanted to let my old political combatant rest in peace. He had died, and I hadn't. In my frayed emotional condition, I felt somehow that Ed Lee and I were both casualties of San Francisco's blood sport.

Lee had begun his career as a young reformer in Chinatown. But decades later, as mayor, he sharply escalated the tech industry takeover of San Francisco. After the mayor pushed through his generous "Twitter tax break" in 2012, many tech corporations (including the social media giant) began moving their headquarters and major satellite offices to San Francisco. Unfortunately, Lee's administration had made no sizable effort to expand the city's limited housing supply for the thousands of tech workers who began pouring into the finite, seven-mile-by-seven-mile metropolis. The predictable housing crunch threw thousands of longtime San Franciscans onto the streets—including many of the artists and activists who had put the city on the world map and many of the teachers, nurses, firefighters, restaurant employees and other workers who were the backbone of the city. None of these bedrock San Franciscans could compete with the earning power of the new tech workforce.

Within the blink of a few years, San Francisco was massively transformed by tech capital and digital culture. Now, riding through the city, there are times I don't know where I am because the distinctive character of a neighborhood has been wiped out, replaced by the anonymous-looking apartment and condo buildings that have been quickly constructed for tech workers, block after block, like stacks of Legos. Meanwhile, cold, sleek skyscrapers—including a gigantic, silver, dildo-like tower—now dominate the downtown skyline, like middle fingers to the city's former human scale. San Francisco now sometimes feels more like a matrix than a living, breathing city.

San Francisco's tech revolution has generated enormous wealth, but its social dislocation has also greatly expanded the ragged armies of the homeless on the streets, creating a starkly divided dystopian city that has turned the once progressive beacon into a cautionary tale. Now leaders in other cities, from

Portland to Philadelphia, worry about becoming "another San Francisco," with grotesque wealth disparities fueled by the rocket blast of digital capitalism.

Early in the tech boom, I began to express my growing sense of loss and alienation about my home city in articles like "How Much Tech Is Too Much?" in *San Francisco Magazine* and in speeches in the lion's lair like one titled "Don't Be a Stanford Dick," which I delivered to a crowded auditorium on the campus known for manufacturing endless ranks of tech bros.

I also wrote a bestselling book that became required civic reading as the 2015 One City One Book selection of the San Francisco Public Library. *Season of the Witch* chronicled San Francisco's tumultuous transformation from a bare-knuckled, foggy port city made for Dashiell Hammett to a free-spirited mecca of poets, musicians, gays, radicals and other outcasts. San Francisco's cultural revolution then crashed under the rainbow gravity of its own excess, a violent conservative backlash and a raging epidemic—only for the city to be reborn as a global beacon of progressive "San Francisco values."

It was a grand urban drama, packed with so many colorful and terrifying incidents and characters that it seemed impossible to have all played out in such a short burst of history in such a relatively small city. Residents of San Francisco—and many more who had bathed in the city's dream light—loved to be told these tales of the city's mythic past. And I loved interviewing the surviving cast members who had starred in San Francisco's legendary pageant and putting their stories on paper.

One reason that *Season of the Witch* was embraced by so many readers under San Francisco's spell was that the city I celebrated was already rapidly disappearing by the time the book was published. The tech boom began shaking the city in the 1990s with the wave of dot-com start-ups, including my own *Salon*. But this entrepreneurial upheaval was nothing compared with the tech earthquake that leveled much of San Francisco's storied past in the second decade of the millennium.

When *Season of the Witch* became a national bestseller, I was invited to speak at libraries, schools, book clubs and civic associations all over the city. Everywhere I was swarmed by people who wanted to tell their own wild stories from San Francisco's past. And many of those who packed these venues were brimming with forlorn San Francisco exit stories, recounting how they had been recently evicted from their homes or were holding on by their fingertips in the overheated housing market. They were using my book to escape into the city's heroic past, when young musicians like Janis Joplin and Jerry Garcia and Marty Balin could pay forty bucks a month to stake out rooms in magnificent, if shabby, Victorian palaces in the Haight-Ashbury neighborhood—now selling to single families for staggering multimillion-dollar prices. These days, that shimmering San Francisco can be seen only in vibrant murals of Janis or Jimi Hendrix or Carlos Santana on walls near pricey espresso bars and artisanal chocolate specialty stores.

During most of my life in San Francisco, I hadn't paid much attention to local politics, smugly confident that progressives with my values were either in power at City Hall or strong enough to keep in check the forces of corporate greed. But as I spoke at countless local book events, I felt the city's ground shifting under my feet. San Francisco no longer felt like the city I had fallen in love with as a teenager during the 1967 Summer of Love, when my family set up residence at the downtown St. Francis Hotel near the Geary Theater, where my father was starring in *The Odd Couple*. As I wrote in the foreword to *Season of the Witch*, that summer "I would trek the city's wind-whipped hills, wander through Chinatown and North Beach, and take the ferryboat to Sausalito. I knew—listening to some older, long-haired teenagers dressed like Moroccan tribesmen, as they played guitars and flutes in a Sausalito square—that I would make San Francisco my home one day." But what do you do, decades later, when your city no longer feels like the enchanted sanctuary with which you once fell in love?

Rumors spread that I was considering a run for mayor in 2015, challenging Mayor Lee, who was widely considered a tool of the tech industry. I was interviewed about the upcoming race by the *San Francisco Chronicle* editorial page chief John Diaz and I didn't rule out the possibility. I began meeting with political advisers to see whether a maverick candidacy like mine would have any chance. The mayoral quest seemed like lunacy, but no major political figure had the nerve to take on Lee and his corporate machine. The mayor began blasting me in media interviews. Ironically I had written admiringly in *Season of the Witch* about a young Ed Lee's beginnings as a crusading tenants' rights lawyer, defending residents of Chinatown projects against predatory landlords and developers. But Lee had since gone to the dark side, aligning himself with the powerful real estate and tech industries that dominated San Francisco.

In the end, I decided not to run for City Hall. My family was opposed to the quixotic crusade, and after everything I had put them through during my *Salon* wild ride, I just couldn't subject them to another ordeal. Like national politics, the San

Francisco electoral arena was becoming increasingly vicious, with the wealthy power brokers around Lee threatening to destroy anyone who challenged him.

I decided instead to play the role of public citizen, using my civic profile as the founder of *Salon* and author of *Season of the Witch* to rally support for progressive city ballot measures and candidates. I threw myself most enthusiastically into the 2015 Board of Supervisors campaign of Aaron Peskin, a sharp-elbowed progressive who already had deep City Hall experience, organizing support for him at a lively literary party at Francis Ford Coppola's Cafe Zoetrope. Mayor Lee and his corporate circle did everything they could to defeat Peskin, whom they realized would become a thorn in the mayor's side as an activist supervisor. But Peskin ran an energetic grassroots campaign and easily prevailed, even winning Lee's Chinatown base.

Why did a man in his mid-sixties who led an increasingly secluded life as a book writer suddenly plunge back into the political maelstrom—even before Donald Trump's triumph made activism an essential public duty? Because I felt my beloved city slipping away—the city where Camille and I had raised our two sons. San Francisco no longer felt like a city where Joe and Nat or their young African-American and Latino friends (none of whom worked in tech) could afford to live, or feel like they belonged. The title of Joe's first dramatic movie—based on the true story of a close childhood friend—said it all: *The Last Black Man in San Francisco*.

———

Ed Lee won his 2015 reelection campaign, but he stirred little enthusiasm at the polls, barely winning a majority of the vote against a field of long-shot and fringe candidates. He had no mandate, and the public outcry about social displacement and the Dickensian gap between rich and poor only grew louder in Lee's new term. Once known as the city of love, San Francisco was now the city of greed. Lee had enough of a memory to sometimes wistfully recall his activist glory days, and enough of a heart to regret what he had become. The growing pressures of his job finally took their toll.

When I came home from the hospital ten days after the mayor's death, I wanted not just my bedroom to be a cocoon from life, but my city. As Camille drove me home, the passing urban scenes seemed more chaotic than ever—they seemed to swirl before my damaged eyes. The streets were clogged with teeming fleets of Uber and Lyft cars, growing congestion that City Hall could not muster the authority to control. The city was shrill and mechanical; a flock of construction cranes hovered monstrously in the skyline. I couldn't make sense of all the loud disorder. There was no warm embrace for me from the city that still had my heart.

Soon after I was released, progressive San Francisco politicians and activists began texting me warm greetings and get-well messages and asking if they could drop by to welcome me home. They were heartfelt salutations to someone they knew might have been suddenly erased from the city's life. But I also felt that my mental and physical status was being tested. Was I ready to rejoin the city's political fray? No; I felt far from combat-ready.

And yet the race to replace the recently departed Mayor Lee was already underway. From my recovery bed, I e-mailed a campaign endorsement to mayoral candidate Jane Kim, a Bernie Sanders–allied local legislator who had fought successfully to make San Francisco City College tuition-free, to offer free local childcare and to raise the minimum wage in the city. Above all, Kim was fighting to protect the many San Franciscans who were in danger of being banished from the city by corporate forces beyond their control. Opposing Kim in the hard-fought, big-spending mayoral race was another supervisor, London Breed, who inherited the corporate patronage that had put Ed Lee in office.

I was in no condition to hit the campaign trail for Kim, but the bugle sounds of political battle were loud enough to penetrate my therapeutic bubble. When she asked me to speak at the campaign rally that kicked off her final sprint to the June 2018 special election, only four months had passed since my hospital release. I was still in speech and physical therapy and I wasn't sure if my words would be intelligible or whether the raucous campaign crowd would make my fragile head spin. But I nervously agreed to appear at the event.

I needed to test my own powers of recovery, to find out whether I could still write a battle-cry speech and have enough vocal strength to deliver it. The mayoral race also felt like a final showdown between progressive San Francisco values and the towering corporate power that poet Allen Ginsberg—gazing at the city's downtown skyline one night many years ago—had described as "Moloch whose eyes are a thousand blind windows . . . whose soul is electricity and banks." How could I not speak out? Or at least *try* to.

The campaign rally was held in a big, barn-like entertainment venue in the South of Market neighborhood. When I arrived to speak, Kim's youthful campaign troops were already hitting the bar. They were dressed in afternoon dance party clothes, while I showed up in a new suit that I had bought for the occasion, one that fit my stroke-diminished body. I immediately felt out of place and out of time, a broken-down political warhorse ready for the pastures.

When it was my turn to speak, my son Nat helped me onto the platform. I wasn't sure I could stand, so I sat awkwardly in a chair and read my speech from pages with enlarged type. It cannot be said that I struck a bold pose on my return to the political arena. But as I began to painstakingly deliver my speech into a hand-held microphone, the boisterous crowd grew quieter, as if straining to hear my words. I explained that I had suffered a stroke several months earlier and begged the audience's patience because "my speech is still a work in progress." And miraculously the crowd that had packed the dance hall to revel in a rowdy pageant of democracy was indeed patient with me, and they gave me enough attention for me to find my rhythm and to hit my high notes about the city we all loved and how we must fight to save its soul.

Five weeks or so later, Jane Kim lost the San Francisco mayoral election to London Breed. Moloch proved too mighty this time. As I've learned many times in my life, politics will break your heart. But staying clear of its ideal-shattering turbulence only invites greater peril. And on those occasions when you do win, the heavens sing and it feels like your city—or your nation—is suddenly within reach of a greatness that makes the mosh pit of democracy seem like it's worth the ordeal.

When you survive a life-shaking medical trauma—especially when I did, around traditional retirement age—you are soon confronted with the epic question: How do I want to enjoy my remaining years, this surprising, final gift of life that has been given to me? And coupled to this is the monumental question, *Where* do I want to live the rest of my life? As we reached our sixties, the "Should we move?" question became increasingly acute for Camille and me. We continually asked ourselves, Have we lost our city; have the corporate cyborgs taken over? Year after year, the do-we-stay-or-do-we-go decision kept getting put off. But having a stroke can really focus the mind.

On the afternoon that I forced myself to climb onstage at the mayoral campaign rally, I knew that my nagging question about where to spend my remaining days was finally answered. When words were still a struggle, San Francisco inspired a passionate eloquence in me. Besides, many of the young people in the campaign crowd that day were tech workers. And yes, the tech industry primarily serves the twin powers of killing and consumerism—i.e., the military and the market. But many of the tech workers pouring into San Francisco these days have more heroic dreams than their corporate overlords—about saving the planet and uplifting humanity.

So there's still hope for San Francisco, even in the age of androids and AI.

Despite the all-too-real depredations of Moloch, I still believe in the fantasy of what the emerald city once was and what it still might become. Despite it all, San Francisco will always be home.

CHAPTER 12

"WHAT FRESH HELL IS THIS?"

Late one summer night, as I was falling asleep in bed, I felt a deep, odd tickling sensation on my back, near my left shoulder blade. It felt like something was squirming under my skin. Indeed it was.

"I think you have a tick bite," Camille announced as she shifted her eyes back and forth between my back and her laptop screen, where she was downloading a flurry of medical pages about blood-sucking arthropods.

"God, no!" I shouted. My head was instantly filled with all the horror stories about tick bites and Lyme disease (and worse) that had been filling my social media pages all summer. "You must be wrong."

"Well, I'm seeing something that's waving eight, tiny striped legs through your skin," she said flatly, clearly trying to quash her own rising panic. "I'm pretty sure it's a tick, and it's burrowed inside you."

A fucking tick! How the hell did one sink its tiny jaws in me? I'm, like, the least outdoorsy person I know. I'm more F. Scott Fitzgerald than Ernest Hemingway. I'm the kind of guy who thinks mountains and forests are best appreciated through a large windowpane while sitting next to a fireplace in a ski lodge, with a warm mug of Irish coffee or a dry martini in hand.

I do love the seashore, however, and I flashed back immediately to the previous weekend we spent at a B&B in Point Reyes, on a quiet Tomales Bay beach. While I was enjoying the sunset on a deck chair one evening, a family of deer broke through a row of nearby bushes, scavenging for food. Deer . . . ticks . . . they go together. Maybe I was bitten in my seashore paradise. But that had been a full week ago. It was more likely that Brando had carried home a little bloodsucker in his lush red fur after roaming the urban wilderness of my neighborhood's Bernal Hill. Are there really ticks in fog-bound San Francisco now?

Because Camille was not certain about how to safely extract the tick, we ended up in the emergency room of St. Mary's Hospital, which is attached to my doctor's office building. It was sometime after midnight on a Saturday night, and the hospital, located near the Haight-Ashbury neighborhood, was hopping. Among other calamities, the busy staff was dealing with two drug overdose cases, including a woman who was tripping on something so jet-fuel powerful that she needed an army of six nurses and orderlies to physically subdue her long enough to inject her with a sedative.

This late-night madness brought back a rush of bad memories for me . . . when my stroke had sent me in darkest night to St. Luke's Hospital's grim emergency chamber. By comparison, the emergency operation at St. Mary's seemed briskly efficient, but I was still filled with anxiety as I waited in a cramped, curtained room to be treated. When a nurse took my blood pressure, he announced it was "kind of high, about 150." No doubt.

Luckily for me, this nurse said he had some experience plucking out ticks with tweezers. And after putting Vaseline on my wound to suffocate the squirming alien, he tweezed it gently out of me by its head, taking care not to crush or rip apart the insect, which could have forced disease-carrying fluids from the tick into my body. The nurse then gave me a pill with a heavy dose of antibiotic to swallow just in case the little bugger carried germs. Lyme disease is not yet as widespread on the West Coast as it is in the East, but the emergency room doctor who popped in to see me said she is treating more tick bites in San Francisco these days. More evidence of nature going mad.

As the weeks passed following my bug-induced trip to the ER, everything seemed fine—no telltale bull's-eye rash on my back or other tick-borne infection symptoms. But I have to say that my stroke has made me feel more physically vulnerable and more prone to freak out about other health scares.

My feeling is, hey, I already paid my dues this year—I don't need to get a fucking tick bite or any other strange affliction. As Dorothy Parker famously and indignantly demanded to know of human existence, "What fresh hell is this?" Maybe this growing level of health concern is a positive development, a sign that I'm recovering from my stroke and I'm reengaging with life. Or maybe it's just the idea of being leeched on by a wriggling, eight-legged creature is too much for me to handle right now. When the nurse proudly pulled the tick's intact head and body out of me, he asked me if I wanted to look at the blood-engorged monster. Um, no thanks.

The truth is, I'd like to keep recovering from my stroke in a protective bubble. After all, I have enough physical woes already, including partial blindness, lingering paralysis and nagging dizziness. Do I really need Lyme disease on top of all that?

But here's the undeniable reality: Life goes on after your stroke, the good, the bad—and in the case of my feasting arthropod, the ugly. Recently I suffered an all-night bout of food poisoning, and who knows what other unpleasant surprises lie in wait for me. Shit happens.

Fortunately, through all my ordeals these past months, major and minor, I'm able to draw on a new sense of inner quiet. After my initial "Oh my God, a tick bite!" freak-out, a soothing calm descended upon me. Even a wry smile about the human comedy. If it's not one thing, it's another!

This is another lesson my stroke has taught me. I'm afraid it's not terribly profound, and you've heard it before. But it rarely seems to sink into us, so I'll add my voice to the chorus. Here's what I deeply know in my heart now. Life is so conditional, so moment to moment. One minute you're fine, and the next your brain feels funny. One second you're here, the next you're not. In the end, if a stroke doesn't finish you off, it might be a tick bite. So live each moment like it's your last, because it just might be.

Embrace your mortality. Even celebrate it. And let the shadow of death make the light in your life only seem brighter.

CHAPTER 13

MAGRITTE AND ME

"**S**ometimes the light's all shining on me, other times I can barely see."

That old Grateful Dead lyric pretty much describes my condition these days, after my stroke wreaked havoc with my visual nerves. How can I put this in medical terms that the average reader will understand? Strokes can really fuck you up. If they don't kill you outright, they generally lay waste to parts of your brain that you're probably going to sorely miss.

So much of our relationship with the world is facilitated by our eyes. You tend to take this for granted, until you don't. We not only take in the world through our eyes; they're the dual portals through which others peer into us and take the measure of our moods and even our souls.

My stroke damaged the neural connection to my left eye, afflicting me with a "gaze palsy" that causes my left pupil to career sharply toward my nose. I can still see out of this eye, sort of—and my right one was mercifully undamaged—but I see double without wearing specially designed spectacles that feature a "smoked glass" effect on half my left lens.

Fortunately I can still read, with some strain. And I can still type, although my right hand remains a heavy and awkward claw because of the lingering paralysis on that side of my body. In general I'm adjusting to whatever disabilities still afflict me. I'm signing checks and paying bills, cleaning the kitchen and taking out the garbage . . . all the daily chores that seemed lost forever in the hospital and will now always seem like miracles to me, instead of dreary tasks.

It's the visual loss that's been hardest for me to adjust to. It's not just the smoked glass in my left lens. I often feel that, due to my visual impairment, I see the entire world through a filmy gauze. Because of my depth perception problems, I am frequently knocking things over in the kitchen. Splat! Oh, shit! That's often the soundtrack as I prepare one of my family meals, which I enjoy doing too much to give up.

Walking on the streets of San Francisco is also a special . . . adventure—particularly when I set out on my own, which I've begun doing lately. Crossing busy streets requires extra nerve, and traffic noise can sound almost deafening because my visual deficit seems to have amplified my auditory senses. Blasting truck horns can make me jump out of my skin. I'm always filled with dread when I read about another pedestrian fatality on San Francisco's increasingly frantic streets—like the beloved pedicab cyclist who was recently the victim of a hit-and-run driver on the city's clogged, chaotic waterfront drive.

When I was in the hospital, our ward was sometimes visited by longtime stroke survivors who volunteered to share their stories. Sometimes they imparted essential advice about adjusting to life on the outside, like ex-cons teaching prisoners about what to expect when they finally get out. One elegantly dressed elderly survivor told us how she overcame her fear of crossing streets when she was released from the hospital. Her sage advice: Never be the first or last to step into the crosswalk. And quickly size up those about to cross the street with you and ask the most amenable-looking one for his or her arm to help you.

Before I cross streets, I have to turn my whole body sharply to the left to see if there's traffic coming from that direction, since I've lost partial vision on my left side. Then I have to warily make the crossing, still twisting awkwardly to my left to make sure there's no car sharply turning the corner into my path or roaring through the red light.

Then there's this additional challenge: If I'm walking toward the sun, the light show effect on my eyes is dazzling, even blinding. I don't have prescription dark glasses yet because the optical lab is still struggling to perfect my indoor glasses. These special spectacles are also expensive, and for some reason known only to the eye-care industry and the federal government, this essential visual aid is not covered by Medicare.

So walking in San Francisco can be a thrilling, heart-pounding experience. These days I feel slower, less nimble than in the past. Like roadkill.

When I used to walk the city streets, dropping into stores and cafés, I prided myself on being friendly, making eye contact and exchanging pleasantries with people—even if I didn't know them. I suppose it was my little way of holding onto San Francisco's warm community feeling, even in today's cold, Darwinian tech environment. Or maybe I'm just an Irish pol at heart.

But now that my left peeper is cockeyed and I wear funny glasses, it makes me self-conscious. When people first look at me close-up, they do a double take. You can see them trying to figure out exactly what is wrong with me. If circumstances permit and I'm in the right mood, I feel compelled to explain to them what happened to me. If not, I just let it ride and all parties, including me, have to let the weirdness hang in the air.

Maybe I'm just being overly sensitive. Over coffee at my corner café, a friend assured me that my new look just gives me "character." But passing people on the streets, I usually can't look them straight in the eye without turning awkwardly to do it. And when I tried to smile during my first months of recovery from paralysis, my crooked grin made it seem like I was smirking at people. I feared some passerby was going to take offense and I would get my ass kicked. *Why are you looking at me weird?!*

I'm not vain, at least not anymore, not at my age. But I always thought of my blue eyes as one of my best features. Now they're a bug, not a feature.

During the initial stroke recovery period, your body is still a work in progress and you can't predict how much of it will rebound as your brain busily searches for new neural pathways to replace the dead ones. By the nine-month mark of my recovery, for instance, my beaming smile had nearly returned to normal. But when I visited my neuro-ophthalmologist around that time, the news was not as good. The doctor informed me that while there might still be some marginal improvement in my left eye, my current condition was pretty much the new normal for me. He did tell me, however, that although the optical nerve damage was permanent, eye surgery might improve my vision by strengthening my eye muscles.

I've made an appointment to meet with the eye surgeon whom he recommended. But I left my doctor's office feeling downcast and in no mood for further medical intervention, especially since surgery always carries some risk and would definitely oblige my poor brain to rewire itself yet again after the operation. As described by my eye doctor, the procedure involves surgically restringing your eye muscles to pull the irises back into alignment—an act of such delicate human origami that it terrifies me.

My worst fear, of course, is that something will go wrong in surgery and my eyesight will actually be further damaged. My vision might not be good today, but I've learned to live (kind of) with its imperfections. Could I navigate through life if I were even more impaired? What if I couldn't even view the premiere of my son Joe's first feature movie, which was selected to screen at the 2019 Sundance Film Festival—a joyous, looming event my family sorely needed? (A few months after I wrote this, Joe's movie, *The Last Black Man in San Francisco*, premiered at Sundance to effusive critical acclaim, and Joe won the festival's Best Director award. Joe's longtime friend, Jimmie Fails, who starred in the film, accepted a Special Jury prize for Creative Collaboration. I did indeed brave the icy streets of Park City, Utah, with my sturdy cane to share in the joy of this miraculous moment in Joe's and Jimmie's lives.)

While I was mulling over these dark thoughts about my vision in the doctor's waiting room, where I was scheduled for another consultation with my eyeglass specialist, a drama suddenly erupted. A man sitting next to me—who seemed almost entirely blind, with dark glasses and a white cane—jumped to his feet in a rage and began yelling. "I should not be made to wait here any longer—I'm not a piece of meat to be left all day in a chair!" Office staff came running to calm him down, but the man clearly had hit his boiling point. I wondered how patient I'd be if I were blind and overlooked.

As I said, I'll meet with the eye surgeon, but I feel inclined not to go through with the procedure, to learn instead to live in my new visual reality. It's true that life now feels once removed to me. But my altered vision can also make my days feel private and interior, even mysterious at times, which is not an unfortunate place to be trapped for a writer.

Coincidentally, around that time I went with a friend to see a major René Magritte exhibit at the San Francisco Museum of Modern Art. I had to stand close to the masterpieces to let my eyes fully appreciate the playful artistry. Museum guards tensed as I stuck my face within inches of each canvas, warning me not to get too close, eyeballing me as closely as I was inspecting Magritte's work.

The show delighted me because the whimsical Belgian surrealist obviously took pleasure in how our eyes can play tricks on us, how there can be a profound gap between what we see and what we perceive. Night can be day in Magritte paintings, a naked woman's beautiful flesh can take on the warm blue shade of the sky, a lush green apple can expand to fill an entire room. Perhaps it was living in a harsh reality—between two world wars and under Nazi occupation—that forced Magritte to seek refuge in his expanded imagination.

If, as Magritte was telling us, the world is filled with infinite meanings, and a distorted sense of reality can produce great art, then my funny, trick-playing eyes can help me see the magic.

CHAPTER 14

TUTTO A POSTO:
THE MEANING OF LIFE . . .
AND DEATH

While I was in the hospital, I was given an advance health care directive form by a family member who has lots of professional experience with these end-of-life protocols. At the time, I found it hard to focus my damaged brain on it. And I think my wife, whose energies were concentrated on helping me live, found the subject too morbid to dwell on. But in the last couple of weeks—ironically, as I got stronger and healthier—I felt a growing urgency to turn my attention to the fateful document. So I recently downloaded the California Advance Health Care Directive form and filled it out.

In case I become too incapacitated to make my own life and death decisions, I granted the power of attorney to my wife, and in case she's unable to make these decisions on my behalf, I empowered two other trusted intimates. While slowly recovering from my stroke, I've become acutely aware of the soap bubble nature of life. And so I left specific instructions in case I suddenly go "pop." I don't want my life prolonged through the miracle (ordeal?) of modern medicine if I'm beyond hope. If, for instance, another stroke turns me into a vegetable. Unless it's eggplant—I love eggplant.

I suppose I'm also thinking more of my eventual end these days because death seems to be in the air. A young man who used to play with my younger son at the nearby playground was shot to death the other afternoon in front of the neighborhood public housing apartment he shared with his mother. The next day Anthony Bourdain was reported to have hanged himself in the bathroom of a five-star hotel in an idyllic Alsatian village while on location for his TV show *Parts Unknown*. A young man clawing to find his place in the city, and an older man who seemed to be on top of the world.

I didn't know Bourdain personally, but like countless others, I felt like I did—and his death had a strangely deep and disorienting effect on me. Bourdain had that gift of making you feel as if you knew him, or convincing you that if you met him, you'd instantly hit it off over drinks at your favorite, weird watering hole. He was roguishly handsome and apparently enjoyed a fantasy love life with a gorgeous and outspoken Italian movie star. He had a dream job that took him to all corners of the big world—an expansive mission that seemed even more essential as our lives became cramped and bordered. He also had an eleven-year-old daughter. People like this are not supposed to kill themselves. And the world felt like it had lost some of its swagger when we needed it most.

We want to believe that our lives tell a story, and that our deaths have a meaning. But all too often they simply seem random. Life is what happens to you while you're busy making other plans, as John Lennon sang. Shortly afterward, he was shot in the head by a complete stranger on the sidewalk outside his apartment building. Tony Bourdain had it all, only he didn't. Sometimes nothing makes sense.

Yet sometimes life—and even death—*do* make sense. David Goodall—the 104-year old Australian scientist who rationally chose to make his final departure a month before Bourdain at an assisted-dying center in Switzerland—made a perfectly understandable, even noble, decision. Goodall had lived a long, satisfying life but was no longer able to enjoy its pleasures because of deteriorating health. Being forced to give up his twin remaining joys—his scholarship and his acting in local theater—were the final blows. His only regrets, Goodall told an intensely curious world press, was that he had lived to be as ancient as he had—and that he had to fly all the way to Switzerland in order to legally die because of Australia's slow-to-change laws about assisted suicide.

How did he want to be remembered, Goodall was asked at a farewell press conference. "As an instrument of freeing the elderly from the need to pursue their life irrespective," he replied. "One wants to be free to choose his death when death is at the appropriate time."

Goodall left this life the way he wanted to, listening to Beethoven's Ninth Symphony. He breathed his last breath with the final note of "Ode to Joy."

Even if life—and death—does seem senseless and out of our control, we can choose to lead our lives as if they have meaning.

It's not just the brilliant and celebrated who teach us how to live and die (or not to). It's the anonymous victims of human horror.

I recently reread this memorable passage from *Man's Search for Meaning*, the brief but monumental book of wisdom by Viktor Frankl, the Austrian neurologist and psychiatrist who survived Auschwitz and Dachau. "We who lived in concentration camps can remember the men who walked through the huts comforting others, giving away their last piece of bread. They may have been few in numbers, but they offer sufficient proof that everything can be taken from a man but one thing: the last of the human freedoms—to choose one's attitude in any given set of circumstances, to choose one's own way."

For most of us, history does not lay waste our lives the way it did to Frankl and his fellow inmates. But no one is spared life's punishments—or its ultimate end. In response to one of my stroke blogs, a friend wrote that sooner or later we're all stricken in one way or the other—she refers to those who haven't been damaged yet as "the temporarily abled."

I was lucky—I had already lived a full life when I was struck in the head at sixty-six like a bolt from heaven. I was already approaching retirement, but it forced a kind of retirement—or redefinition—on me. Every morning I wake up, I inventory myself, to remind me of what I've lost physically, what I've recovered and what will probably never come back. Then I try to realistically assess what I can do that day and the next, on my own or with the help of others. I felt entombed by my stroke. Now I'm coming back to life; but, finally, I will be entombed again.

Choosing my attitude toward life: That's the only real power I have, as Frankl observed. There are moments when I give in to self-pity, foul moods and bitter regret. Why was I locked into such a stressful life? Why did I choose such a combative and financially unstable career as dissident journalism? Why didn't I lose weight and learn to meditate *before* I had a stroke? Some of these life decisions were under my control, of course—but some of the directions I took in life were my fate.

In any case, I quickly realized it was up to me how I wanted to carry my wounded self through the rest of my life—with a heavy sense of loss, or with a lightness that can lift my family's burden and others in my wider community. As I said, it's easy to dwell on my physical disabilities; I must now live within these limitations every day of my life.

But I'm still living on this Earth and I choose to treat that as the miracle it is. And, as a result, I allow a giddy joy to spread through my soul—and to let it astonish and please others, who expect, perhaps, a more hobbled and tragic me. Even if they fear my new goofiness might be related to my stroke, so what? Fuck it, let my freak flag fly.

This explosion of light within me doesn't erase death's long shadow. This darkness is a slowly growing presence in my life. But preparing for my end is not a morbid exercise for me. I feel compelled to keep reassuring my wife of this—and other people who love me. This death planning makes me feel that I'm getting my life in order, even when there is so little to life or death that is predictable and orderly.

There's an Italian expression, *tutto a posto*, which comes to mind—everything's OK, everything is in its proper place. That's what I'm after these days, even if the goal is illusory.

Lately I've been gathering boxes of research materials from my various book projects—boxes that are now stored in my office and basement. I'm preparing to give away these research materials to institutions where hopefully they'll enjoy a longer shelf life than I will. I'm being helped by Karen Croft, my collaborator on all my book projects. An ardent Italophile, Karen was the one who explained to me the meaning of *tutto a posto*. We started by filling cardboard boxes with taped interviews, transcripts and archival treasures from our work on *Season of the Witch,* which we decided to donate to the History Center at the downtown San Francisco Public Library—an obvious choice because we did much of the book's research there, aided by the knowledgeable and helpful staff.

The book explored San Francisco's convulsive history, from the 1967 Summer of Love to the AIDS epidemic's reign of terror in the 1980s. By examining my beloved hometown's recent past, I sought to understand how the human imagination can liberate an entire city (and then tantalize the world)—with enough collective effort and fairy dust. Karen and I taped hours and hours of interviews with members of the Grateful Dead, Jefferson Airplane, Big Brother and the Holding Company, the Diggers, the San Francisco Mime Troupe, the leaders of the city's gay revolution, San Francisco 49ers living legends, veteran city cops, aging radical lawyers, politicians, poets and dreamers . . . all of whom rebuilt San Francisco to correspond with their dreams. All of this precious storytelling now has the right home, in the reader-friendly rooms of the main San Francisco Public Library's sixth-floor History Center. *Tutto a posto.*

Choosing where to donate our boxes of research material from our books *Brothers* and *The Devil's Chessboard* is more complicated because this history chapter—the Kennedy brothers' martyrdom and the national security intrigue behind their violent deaths—is so terribly fraught. What about the John F. Kennedy Presidential Library in Boston, where Karen and I did much of our research on both books? We reached out to the library through a friend in the Kennedy family. But the JFK Library is controlled more by the National Archives than it is by the family, and so it's subject to all the murky political and bureaucratic forces flowing through Washington, D.C.

We're sitting on a historical treasure trove, including rare taped interviews with prominent members of the inner Kennedy circle who spoke with us late in life with cathartic honesty about what they believe the Kennedy brothers were trying to accomplish, what really happened to them and why. The names in our files of revealing interviews include Senator Edward Kennedy, Robert McNamara, Theodore Sorensen, Arthur Schlesinger Jr., Richard Goodwin, Edwin Guthman, Nicholas Katzenbach, Adam Walinsky and Frank Mankiewicz—dozens of historical names and less-known political players, nearly all of them now dead.

It was Karen who urged me to interview these Kennedy New Frontier men and women before they all passed away. We both knew they had a story to tell about this dark American tragedy, a deeper story that had become lost in the mists of Camelot. And now, what will be the final resting place of their ghostly words, their unspeakable stories about the lives and deaths of the Kennedy brothers? We're still waiting to hear if the Kennedy Library will make room in its archives and program schedule for this disturbing history.

All of this packing up of audiotapes, government documents and rare books—it's part of getting my life in order. It's another

TUTTO A POSTO

kind of advance directive. Like all historians, I hoped that my years of work would in some way change history—would shift America's understanding of the epic Kennedy drama. Will my work as a journalist and historian finally get mainstream acknowledgment? Not in my lifetime. I can concede this now, even though I firmly believe that Karen and I essentially solved both Kennedy assassinations. It's all right; as Karen likes to say, the work was its own reward.

But if our work didn't rewrite history, I know that it affected many readers, including some of those with whom we spoke who had been closest to the Kennedy brothers. I like to think that reading our books gave these men and women some clarity and comfort before they died.

During my interview with Ted Sorensen, JFK's close aide and poetic speechwriter, he told me, "If I could know that my friend of eleven years died as a martyr to a cause, that there was some reason, some purpose why he was killed—and not just a totally senseless, lucky sharpshooter—then I think the whole world would feel better." Reading our books and other revisionist histories of the Kennedy era—like James Douglass's *JFK and the Unspeakable*—finally gave Sorensen and other Kennedy intimates this reassurance. That John and Robert Kennedy had indeed lived and died for a greater reason.

Looking back at my long years of research and writing, that's meaning enough for me.

CHAPTER 15

ALL THINGS MUST PASS

None of us knows how and when she or he is going to die. But after having my stroke, I began to think I'd be finished off at some point by another stroke. This fatal possibility was driven into me while I was still recuperating in my hospital stroke ward by the medical staff, who stressed during patient meetings that our chances of having a second stroke were even higher unless we reduced our risk factors. The numbers tell the stark story: Of the nearly 800,000 people who suffer strokes each year, almost 200,000 of them have already been stricken at least once before.

Fortunately I am now leading a healthier life. Since my stroke nine months ago, I've shed close to forty pounds, slashed my systolic blood pressure numbers from a high of 170 to around 125, started taking a baby aspirin every day (to reduce my chances of forming another blood clot), and decompressed my life through meditation, exercise and stopping to smell the roses.

I feel lit up inside every day by a golden glow, a warm, bright realization that starts spreading in me soon after I wake up. My very first thought each morning upon surfacing from sleep is, Wow, I'm fucked up, I've had a stroke, my eyes and limbs don't quite work right. And then, in a rush, I immediately think, Damn, I'm still *here*. I can move my body and get out of bed. I can make breakfast!

And yet a shadow of death still flutters nearby me, rustling darkly at different moments throughout my day. After all, a small part of my brain died during my stroke, when the blood clot cut off oxygen to it. Part of me is already dead. And that's the way I sometimes feel—like I have one foot in the grave. Death looms closer in my life nowadays, despite all my new health and vitality. Despite the fact that, with my reduced risk factors, I'm probably less likely to die from another stroke than I am from getting hit by the proverbial truck on the increasingly deranged streets of San Francisco.

To tell you the truth, I've dwelled on death and dying ever since I was a boy. Maybe it was because I had an older father— he was fifty when I was born, much older than other parents in those years. I was always worried my dad would keel over. It turned out I had nothing to worry about. He lived to be a ripe old ninety-four.

But I was an anxious kid. Life's fragility and other morbid thoughts consumed me.

I became anorexic when I was twelve, and my spirit began fading away as my flesh disappeared. I felt half-alive—a strange, dizzy sensation of partial existence that returned to me after my stroke. Looking back, I think I was slowly vanishing myself because, on the cusp of adolescence, I wasn't sure I wanted to join the cold, cruel grown-up world. It was a hunger strike against adult life. I could immediately relate to the Who song "My Generation" when it came out not long after, with its powerful punch line: "Hope I die before I get old." But as I was slowly starving myself to death, I finally made a conscious decision to live. I remember the evening with sharp clarity. I rose slowly from my bed, like it was a coffin, drifted to the kitchen, took an Oreo cookie from a package in the cupboard and devoured it. It tasted like life. It was the first solid food I'd had in months.

I'm now sixty-six years old. I've lived a long, robust life—a life close to what I wanted and imagined. I've survived, for now, what could have been a fatal medical trauma. And these days I find myself singing from the songbook of Leonard Cohen, the late master of darkly funny irony: "Tonight will be fine . . . for a while."

For a while. All of our lives are conditional, are moment to moment. But somehow that overwhelming reality no longer overwhelms me. Life and death have become bed partners. The lion lies down with the lamb.

Now that I've made peace with death, my soul is tranquil enough to prepare for my final exit. I find myself reading about the final days of those whose lives I've admired. How did they greet the final unknown? What wisdom or insight, if any, did they impart as they drew their last breaths?

Lately I've become obsessed with George Harrison's death. The spiritual Beatle departed this life in 2001 at age fifty-eight,

ALL THINGS MUST PASS

succumbing to cancer after a lifetime of smoking. Like millions in my generation, I followed the Beatles' lead through my early life—the magical mystery tour through drugs, spiritual exploration, love's blossoming, political awakening and more. The "deep Beatles"—George and John—made a special impact on me. So it made sense to me, following my stroke, that I should look to my early mentors for clues, for a kind of direction when it comes to end-of-life questions.

In Lennon's case, death came violently and unexpectedly on the sidewalk outside his New York apartment building in December 1980. There was no chance to grow old and to muse about the final stage of life—which is a shame because I was among the countless Beatles fans who loved reading John's raw, introspective commentary about life, love, music and the great quest for human liberation in *Rolling Stone* magazine and other media venues. I'm sure his self-examination about the meaning of life and death would have been just as enlightening if he'd been allowed to live longer.

Weirdly, George too nearly died at the hands of a deranged fan, a man who broke into his Friar Park mansion in 1999 and stabbed him nearly to death. George, who had been preparing for death most of his life, was serenely giving himself over to fate in the midst of the brutal attack. But his wife, Olivia, decided it wasn't yet his time to go, and she broke a lamp over the attacker's head.

As a result, George had nearly two more years to get ready for his great transition.

The final years were not easy for George as his cancer spread from his lungs to his brain and he pursued various medical treatments around the world. But in the end, he was ready to die, meeting with those he loved and with whom he had made musical history, and consoling them instead of the other way around.

"We held hands," recalled Paul McCartney, who visited with George—the bandmate he called his "baby brother"—at a New York area hospital shortly before his death. "It's funny, even at the height of our friendship—as guys—you would never hold hands. It just wasn't a Liverpool thing. But it was lovely."

For a heavenly being, George was very much of this world, thoroughly enjoying his fill of those life pleasures offered to a rock star. As a devout disciple of the Krishna Consciousness movement, he gave himself over to long bouts of chanting and meditation. But besides the "bag of prayer beads," recollected Ringo Starr, George also carried around "this big bag of anger." His inner fury and wicked humor were on scorching display in songs like "Taxman" and "Piggies." He might have strived mightily to transcend this material world, but this son of the Liverpool working class—his father drove a school bus—truly hated handing over the lion's share of his new riches to the British welfare state. ("Now my advice for those who die/Declare the pennies on your eyes." Like I say, wicked.)

I love both sides of George. I understand his contradictions. George's religion required no denial of rock stardom. But George was a deep enough soul to recognize its limits, to see that no amount of sex or drugs could bring him the bliss he sought.

No popular artist did more to spread the wisdom of Eastern religion to the West—or a haunting sense of the ineffable—than George Harrison. At age fifteen, when I first absorbed the meaning of "Within You Without You"—pulsing hypnotically

ALL THINGS MUST PASS

on the *Sgt. Pepper's Lonely Hearts Club Band* album to the exotic drone of a sitar and tabla—it took me somewhere deep inside myself that I didn't know existed: "When you've seen beyond yourself then you may find / Peace of mind is waiting there . . ."

There are times even now that I think I only must listen to George's music to help me prepare for death.

George was too cool to hustle his religion, but it clearly imbued everything he did. The spiritual aura around him was strong enough in February 1968 to draw the other Beatles and their shining retinue—including various lovers, Mia Farrow and her younger sister (Dear Prudence) and fellow musicians Donovan Leitch and Mike Love—to the remote ashram of the Maharishi Mahesh Yogi in the foothills of the Himalayas. This enchanted retreat, which lasted several weeks and gave the Beatles a unique respite from the media madness of celebrity, took the group to a higher creative plane. They wrote nearly all of their final masterpiece, *The White Album,* among the fragrant jasmine, emerald-green parrots and mischievous monkeys of the Maharishi's lush compound.

This blaze of creativity could never have been accomplished without George's inner light. Only George could have heard his guitar gently weeping as he strummed its strings outside an ashram bungalow.

The principal reason George did not fear death was that he believed life was only a transitory shadow existence. Death was no more than shedding "one suit and putting on another," George said. A believer in reincarnation, he prayed that death would release him from millennia of birth, death and rebirth and because of his spiritual achievements he would finally be liberated from this mortal coil and achieve nirvana. I have no doubt that the Beatles were bodhisattvas who came to earth to help take humanity to a higher level. George, at last, deserved to be "free from birth."

When he knew he was close to death, George felt he could not depart this world at his Friar Park estate, which he feared would become a media circus and attract the kind of madness that had come shrieking into his home at knifepoint two years earlier. So, fearing for the safety of his wife, Olivia, and son, Dhani, he asked his friend, security expert Gavin de Becker, to allow him to die at de Becker's gated estate in Los Angeles. As he prepared to leave this existence, George was surrounded by Olivia, Dhani and two longtime fellow Krishna devotees, who chanted and prayed with him.

In the 2011 documentary about George made by Martin Scorsese, Olivia described the moment her husband stopped breathing: "There was a profound experience that happened when he left his body. It was visible. Let's just say that you wouldn't need to light the room if you were trying to film it. He just . . . lit the room." Dying light. It's a phenomenon that many palliative caregivers remark upon as they help the dying in their final moments. It comes as no surprise that George gave off this radiance as his spirit floated away.

As I've remarked before, I'm not a religious man. I have not led a life remotely as spiritual as someone like George Harrison. But purely instinctually I believe in a human spirit that outlasts our lives. And I believe that beautiful music—transcendent music— helps us feel this other, more sublime existence. All of us who love the Beatles' music are more divine for being transported by it.

ALL THINGS MUST PASS

Come to think of it, maybe instinct is not the only reason I believe in an afterlife.

The first time I saw the Beatles' American debut album, *Meet the Beatles*, I was walking as a boy with my mother, Paula, past the local record store window in Studio City, where the album cover was being displayed. Catching sight of the mop-tops, she laughed. "Now there are four faces that only a mother could love." But my mother was a singer and loved music—and she came to fall in love with beautiful Beatles songs like "Yesterday," "And I Love Her" and "Here, There and Everywhere."

My mother came fully to life with her children. She once told my sister Cindy that before she had kids, she sometimes woke up feeling empty and desolate. After she became a mother, she said, she never felt that way again. My mother was a producer of life, and we four kids were the show she was constantly staging.

Paula was only sixty when she died. The first stroke didn't kill her. She was slowly recovering from that one when the second stroke hit. Each stroke thereafter took more from her until the final one. I was on vacation in Hawaii with Camille, then my wife-to-be, when my mother died in San Francisco. I felt the moment she stopped breathing, like a flash of lightning to my heart. I turned to Camille in bed and told her something awful had just happened.

When we returned to San Francisco, I dropped by the Opera Plaza apartment where we were going to move my elderly father, to make sure it was ready for him. I was looking around the living room when some movement down the short hallway to the bedroom caught my eye. I thought someone from the apartment building staff was making some final arrangements in the bedroom, and I stopped and gazed down the hallway. I saw instantly who it was, and it neither shocked nor frightened me. It was broad daylight, and I was perfectly clearheaded. My mother was there, walking in the bedroom. And I knew exactly why she was there. She had to make sure the new apartment was right for my aging father, the bedroom where he would die a few years later, as my family and I kept vigil.

I don't believe in ghosts, but I know what I saw that afternoon. And I feel that George is somehow right. This life is not the end of the story. All things must pass. But when we do, we have an unknown destination.

CHAPTER 16

CIRCLE OF LOVE

Recovering from a stroke is a lonely, soul-testing ordeal. But it also can be an intensely social experience, sweeping up family members, friends, ex-lovers, old work colleagues, former classmates, medical personnel, physical therapists, health insurance bureaucrats and random strangers in its mighty, relentless tide. I don't want to say it takes a village—because I'm a confirmed big-city boy, and I think of small towns as nests of weird intrigue, petty grievances and compulsory rituals. But it *does* take what I prefer to call "a circle of love" to become whole again, or at least some new version of being alive.

I get this expression from a silly game that my extended family began playing whenever we found ourselves in a pool on vacation, "The Circle of Love." The game—which became a favorite of our two sons during their childhood and of many cousins, aunts and uncles—involves hitting a beach ball back and forth in a pool circle as many times as possible without letting it splash down into the water. Since we're stats-conscious sports fans, we count out loud each successful volley as the colorful orb is propelled back into the air by outstretched fingertips. But we're all on the same team—we're working together to keep the big ball in flight for as long as we can. The only competition is with wind and gravity.

A sudden catastrophe like a stroke can make or break this circle of love. I was lucky—mine only became tighter during my five weeks in the hospital, and has remained durable ever since. Camille stopped work for over a year to help care for me. I can no longer drive because my eyesight is askew, so for weeks and months she ferried me to most of my medical and physical therapy appointments. She drives a new Prius I bought for us just before my stroke, a car I'll never again pilot. When I get in the passenger seat, she's often listening to the Beatles channel on Sirius XM. *Baby you can drive my car.* We suddenly found ourselves so often together—after three decades of marriage with our share of joy and rough strife—that we began calling my recovery our second honeymoon.

Joined at the hip together throughout my rehab drama, Camille and I developed a sick sense of humor to get us through it all. She too is a writer, now working on a book that artfully raises a nineteenth-century bohemian marriage from its dusty tomb. So she and I entertain each other during all the medical waiting room tedium by coming up with book titles for today's modern stroke victims—no, not *victims,* we're supposed to call ourselves stroke *survivors* these days. In that relentlessly positive vein, we started plotting out a book modeled on those upbeat hospital guides they hand out to you—we called it, *Congratulations . . . You're Having a Stroke!*

The truth is that this recuperation regimen really did bind us tighter, at a time when many marriages are wearing out. My stroke had left me "bruised and battered . . . unrecognizable to myself," as Springsteen sang. But Camille still knew me. She kept reminding me who I was. When I felt unlovable and beyond love, when I felt like I was the subject of a cruel medical experiment, she hugged me tightly in my hospital bed, and I felt that I could live another day.

My sister Cindy, a doctor in Portland, Oregon, also appeared when I most needed her, conferring with my stroke ward doctors and making sure I was getting proper treatment. She spent one of the early, frightening nights in my hospital room, sleeping on a cot and talking softly with me late into the night like we were still two kids falling asleep together. Cindy flew down to look after me even though she was burdened with her own health troubles. Weeks later she would undergo heart surgery for atrial fibrillation—recurring sieges of irregular heartbeats that left her breathless and exhausted.

My sister has a habit of showing up in the middle of family medical emergencies just when it's most critical, providing expert advice and reassurance that it's OK to question doctors and nurses about a loved one's hospital care. When you're sprawled half-conscious in a hospital bed, you need someone you trust to advocate for you. "Don't you think he should be cathed every four hours instead of six? Can the dosage on this medicine be

CIRCLE OF LOVE

reduced, since it makes him so dizzy?" You know, that kind of polite but diligent hospital bedside supervision.

Margaret, my other sister, also swooped into my hospital—from her home in Washington, D.C.—bringing her usual warm and giddy sense of humor, which I desperately needed. Embracing the absurdity in life and its never-ending travails—and even getting dark laughs from it—has been essential to my recovery. And my sister shares this screwy sense of humor.

As I noted earlier, when my new life felt too sad and weird, I sometimes escaped into my two alter egos. These new split personalities were also born out of my desire to make Margaret and Camille, who are the best of friends, laugh—and to create an absurd fantasy world as a refuge from reality. One of my new alter egos, "Strokey," was a bit nutty—he was always ready to spring out of bed in the hospital before he was quite ready. He's a can-do guy, even when he clearly can't do. And "Nigel," you might recall, is a charming English chap who's always *"ever* so grateful" for the smallest of kindnesses. Even when a nurse came to stab me with another blood-thinning shot in my already black-and-blue belly, I would suddenly morph into Nigel, who would profusely thank the bewildered woman: "Oh, you've been *ever* so kind to me! How can I *ever* repay you?"

My brother, Steve, also stood sentry by my hospital bedside, and in the months since I've returned home we've fallen into a pleasant Friday afternoon ritual, strolling on the fire trail that winds its way up nearby Bernal Hill, with my dog, Brando, tagging along. We talk about family, politics and movies—the Talbot clan's holy trinity. And our conversation takes unexpected detours into corners of our childhood that sometimes I've forgotten, or only half-remember.

Like the time Steve thought it would be a swell idea to follow behind in our mailman's footsteps and swipe any interesting-looking packages he left in our neighbors' mailboxes. We were determined to find a gift for our mother and shopping at Macy's was beyond our abilities. As I recall, we did discover a pair of black stockings in one neighbor's mailbox, as we merrily looted the packages that the mailman delivered on his route. But when we proudly presented the silky lingerie to our mother, our racket quickly unraveled. Our poor father, after arriving home from a long day on *The Ozzie and Harriet Show* set, had to go door to door with our pilfered booty and apologetically return the stuff to our neighbors. I would love to know how he explained why those black stockings had fallen into his hands.

Only my sisters and brother can still connect me to the earliest mad capers and murky memories of my life. But following my stroke, my circle of love has expanded wider than my family. I was the beneficiary of many random acts of kindness early in my recovery. When lay ministers dropped by my hospital room or psychology interns or acupuncture students who sought to use my body for training, I was always glad to see them. In my condition, any laying on of hands was welcome. And sometimes these strangers provided just the small touch of inspiration that I needed to get through the day. It wasn't the religious lessons or therapeutic nostrums that often came with their visits. It was their willingness to drop by a complete stranger's room on the stroke ward, never knowing what sort of human tragedy was about to confront them.

I remember the young man in his mid-thirties who suddenly showed up in my hospital room late one afternoon. He walked with a cane and his speech had the slightest slur, remnants of the stroke that had almost killed him at age twenty-nine. Months later, I still remember the story he told. The oldest son of a tight-knit working-class family that lived on the Avenues in San Francisco, he had been his parents' bright star on the rise. Management job at a city bank branch office, founder of a sports charity, regular seats at the San Francisco Giants ballpark as the team was driving for its first World Series championship in 2010. And then the blinding headache as he was lying in bed one evening. It's the last thing he remembered before falling into a coma that lasted four weeks. By the time he awoke, the Giants had completed their impossible post-season victory run. Family members, astounded by his sudden awakening, had to tell him what he missed.

And then came the inevitable depression, "darkness visible," in the words of William Styron. He had awakened to an entirely new life. He was no longer able to work as a bank manager; he had to hand over the sports charity to his brother. He began losing his life force and found it harder and harder to get out of bed each day. His parents grew worried about him, and to cheer him up, his father took him one evening to see a Golden State Warriors basketball game. But he had gained weight during his recovery and it was difficult for his slight, aging father to push his wheelchair up the long ramp to the stadium.

The young man felt humiliated; he was furious at himself. He knew he had to change his life or continue dying slowly. The next morning, he pulled himself out of bed, grabbed his cane and headed on wobbly legs for the front door, to do laps on the sidewalk outside. His father was terrified for him and ran behind his unsteady son with the wheelchair. But he made it unassisted to the street corner that day. And each day he ventured a little farther, aided by his family and their unwavering love.

He had arrived at my hospital room that day by bus—a trek that entailed switching routes mid-journey. In my still-hazy condition, I marveled that any stroke survivor could manage to navigate bustling, steep San Francisco by bus. My visitor loomed like Magellan before me.

But he told his story without any pride or embellishment. I had to entice it out of him in my usual journalistic way of making conversation. Once upon a time he'd sped in the fast lane; now he got around on a cane and by bus. But there was no self-pity in his voice. He was helping people who needed to hear his story, who needed to hear that everything might be different, but there is still life after a stroke. Maybe the purpose of his life had even grown after his stroke.

During my recovery, I have found that some survivors' change-of-life stories thrill me, while others send me spinning downward to the pits of gloom. It's not that I need sugar-coating—in fact, relentlessly upbeat stories just seem silly and annoying. They bring out the cynical journalist in me—I want to poke holes in their chirpy patter. But I always find myself responding to personal accounts that have a truthful mix of shadow and light. Stories that have the right existential tone. "You must go on, I can't go on, I'll go on," in the absurd wisdom of Samuel Beckett.

My stroke landed its blow shortly before Thanksgiving. As I write this, fall is coming again, earlier this year in San Francisco. The air is chilled; it's Mary Poppins windy. But one afternoon, I got it into my Toad-like head that I had to walk up Bernal Hill for exercise. In my wobbliness, I felt that I could've been blown away by the gales rushing down at me as I struggled up the steep grade. But my son Nat quickly took me by the arm. He was beset by his own woes at the time and they absorbed us both as we walked together. But his grip was strong and effortless. He's built sturdy, like a wrestler. His muscled arms are covered in tattoos—he already looks like the chef he's training to become. His flesh art is a canvas of San Francisco and family history: the city in flames during the 1906 earthquake, his grandfather's '55 Oldsmobile, a picture of his beautiful grandmother around the time she was a World War II Rosie the Riveter. He has a new tattoo—a Chinese food takeout carton emblazoned with the slogan he hopes will guide his cooking career: "Everybody eats." Nat has a big heart.

"That's OK, Dad, I got you," he said, as I wavered in the wind.

THE FUTURE'S NOT OURS TO SEE

O n the exact one-year anniversary of my stroke, I found myself huddled in a cramped hotel room in Carmel, California, with Camille, Nat, his friend Dylan and our dog, Brando. We were fleeing the relentless clouds of smoke and ash from California's latest wildfires, which had consumed the entire town of Paradise in the Sierra foothills and left a deadly pall hanging over the Bay Area, more than one hundred miles away. Day after day, the streets of San Francisco looked otherworldly, with even the tallest buildings and hills disappearing in a thick, yellow-gray haze, and people wearing face masks like the whole city was an intensive care ward. It was eerily quiet because the dangerously polluted air had forced the closure of all schools. There were no kids playing in parks or playgrounds, and most people had shut themselves inside their homes or offices with the windows closed.

San Francisco was now plagued with some of the deadliest air in the world, rivaling the most polluted cities in China and India. Public health authorities were warning it was "no place for old men" or other living things—especially those with a history of respiratory disease (like me). The incidence of strokes and heart attacks was also spiking in the Bay Area. So after more than a week of living under confinement and trying not to breathe too deeply while running essential errands, we decided to pack up and head for Carmel—one of the few communities within driving distance of San Francisco where the air was listed as "moderately healthy."

Carmel was a little smoke-free oasis hugging the ocean, with a patch of gloriously blue sky overhead. The white sand beach—which I remembered in Carmel's more conservative past as heavily posted with signs full of stern dos and don'ts—was packed with giddy refugees and their cavorting dogs, all breathing more freely in the clean sea air. We had apparently booked the last dog-friendly hotel room in town, at movie legend Doris Day's Cypress Inn, an adobe hacienda not far from the beach. To our surprise, we were informed at the check-in counter that Hollywood's tomboyish sweetheart was still alive at ninety-six and still mad for her dogs—which is why Brando was treated like his celebrity namesake by the cheery hotel staff, and even served food in a brightly colored dog bowl in the hotel lobby. (Sadly, the legendary actress has since passed on.)

Despite the staff's conviviality, which seemed to mirror Doris Day's own bubbly screen persona, the mood in the crowded hotel lobby was somber and edgy. People perched on stuffed sofas or squeezed into standing-room-only spaces, clutching drinks from the bar and swapping stories of frantic escapes and toxic air. Even the hotel guests' dogs, which ran the gamut from bony Chihuahuas to burly huskies, seemed emotionally exhausted as they lay quietly on the lobby floor, next to a baby grand piano and—ironically—a roaring fireplace.

The hotel lounge singer poised next to the piano player gamely tried to pick up people's spirits, but it sounded like her heart wasn't in it as she sang of "blue skies, nothing but blue skies from now on."

We weren't certain if her song selection was intentionally ironic.

In the bar area, the piped-in Doris Day song "Que Será, Será"—from her uncharacteristically intense role in the Hitchcock thriller *The Man Who Knew Too Much*—sounded more to the point. "Whatever will be will be, the future's not ours to see."

The lyrics summed up the anxious but weirdly carefree mood in the jammed hotel, filled with old Hollywood nostalgia artifacts, ceramic statues and paintings commemorating dearly departed poodles, and exiles from California's growing climate apocalypse. The hotel felt like a sanctuary, but a make-believe one. Outside, you could see the plumes of smoke drifting over the Santa Cruz Mountains in the far distance. This was "the new abnormal," as Governor Jerry Brown described the state's fiery reality.

There wasn't enough space in our hotel room for the five of us, but there was no way we could leave Dylan behind in the smoke-choked city. He was temporarily living in his van, and his life was too exposed to the elements. That night, we ate at a Japanese-Californian restaurant called the Flying Fish

Grill. It wasn't exactly dog-friendly, but they couldn't turn Brando away when I shuffled inside on my cane, precariously hanging on to his leash.

Over steamed California artichoke appetizers with Japanese-inflected dipping sauces, we talked about the kitchen arts that Nat was learning at the San Francisco Cooking School. While growing up, Nat had watched me turn out countless family meals. But now his culinary skills were exceeding mine and I was ready to hand him the frying pan. It was a night for reflection, and I reminded Nat that when he was growing up, our two favorite pastimes as a family were going to restaurants and going to movies. Now one of our two sons was making movies, and the other one was training to be a chef, with a plan to open his own uniquely San Franciscan eating joint.

"Your mom and I have succeeded as parents!" I proclaimed with a laugh, but I surprised myself by meaning it. The truth is that Camille and I constantly worried we were blowing it as parents, because neither of our sons had followed a conventional educational path. But somehow they had figured out where they were going.

My tablemates then raised a toast to the one-year landmark of my survival. But I suddenly felt weirdly out of sorts—dizzy, headachy, awkward. Eating dinner, I bit my tongue hard enough to make it gush blood—something I hadn't done since early in my recovery, when my facial muscles were more lethargic. It wasn't just the morbid anniversary that was disorienting me; it was the mournful sense that the world was on fire, and instead of a wise leader chosen by history to confront this existential challenge, we had a mad emperor in Washington who was fiddling while the planet burned.

Once upon a time, I threw myself into these epic human struggles, to fight war, injustice, environmental destruction. And the global climate crisis was the most colossal crucible of my aging life. But now age sixty-seven, still enfeebled by my stroke, I felt too old and weak, my spirit insufficient to the great task at hand. These days, I often wanted to escape into an old Hollywood movie with a happy ending, even a preposterous Doris Day–Rock Hudson fade-out.

The next morning, before we headed back to the still-smoky city, we took Brando for one final romp on the beach. The long curve of white sand was again a cacophonous panorama of barking animals and frolicking humans, all of them discharging a frantic energy as if they had just been let out of a kennel. It made sense to me that this end-of-world scene was being played out not just "on the beach," like the post-apocalyptic 1959 movie, but on a beach overrun by dogs. Heaven will surely be dog-friendly.

A white-haired woman was strolling along the bluff overlooking the sand and surf with her small, fluffy dog. She began chatting with Camille in that easy way that dog owners do. She had just arrived in Carmel after driving all the way from a Los Angeles suburb that was also on fire. The Golden State was aflame, from north to south. As humans, dog-lovers tend to be better bred—more social and empathetic, if sometimes endearingly nutty. The woman told Camille that her small dog was blind but she liked to bring him to dog-friendly beaches so he could smell and hear his fellow canines as they barked and splashed in the surf. She said it made him happy. I could relate—I'm now nearly half blind too, and crazy canine carnivals like the one spinning out of control on the beach make me laugh out loud like a kid.

163

When we arrived back home in San Francisco, the air still smelled like a dying campfire. But as I slept that night, I was awakened by a soft pelting noise on our bedroom window, one that I hadn't heard for so long that it took me a moment to recognize what it was. Rain! The beginning of a stormy season that would wash the sky clean and soak bone-dry Northern California on and off for the next several months.

The morning newspaper was filled with stories about the fresh-faced pack of Democrats who had won Congressional seats in the 2018 midterms against daunting obstacles, even in districts that had been cynically carved out to favor Republicans. It was an incoming political class led by women and encompassing the full racial, ethnic, religious and sexual rainbow of America. The halls of Washington were suddenly filled with their gushing energy and idealism.

I can't help it, I was born and raised in Hollywood—I was made to believe in happy endings. My life has had many of them. Besides, I'm the father of two young men, so I have to believe in the future.

After breakfast, I found myself clicking on "Feeling Good"—the Nina Simone version:

> *"It's a new dawn, it's a new day, it's a new life for me*
> *Oh, and I'm feeling good"*

I like the Nina Simone interpretation because it's far from sugary. In her throaty, sharply enunciated voice, her joy sounds hard-won. She sounds like we deserve to celebrate because, despite all odds, we're still here.

SONGS FOR STROKEYS: A DANCE AND MEDITATION LIST FOR STROKE THRIVERS

The four songs that meant the most to me after my stroke, and that made me want to dance with the most defiant exuberance, were:

- **"ALIVE,"** by Pearl Jam. I kept watching the black-and-white video on YouTube for obvious reasons, shouting out the chorus (as best as I could with my constricted voice box): "Oh-oh, I'm still alive!" Goddamn right.

- **"I'M NOT LIKE EVERYBODY ELSE"** (*that's* for sure), by the eternally impish and adorable Kinks.

- **"IT'S ALL IN MY MIND,"** by the venerable Scottish bar band Teenage Fanclub, which kickstarts with these lyrics: "I was in the water, I was half a human." Which accurately describes my mental state some days.

- **"I NEVER LOVED A MAN (THE WAY I LOVE YOU),"** by Aretha Franklin, especially the slow, sinuous, sexy version the Queen of Soul performed during her late 1960s concerts. Because strokeys sometimes need deep inspiration to get back their groove. I found the best live version of this song on YouTube the day after Aretha ascended to heaven, in which the elegant goddess works up a sweat, to the eye-popping excitement of the young European men hugging her stage.

Here's the rest of my dance list, a Top Fifty (or so), in no particular order—because, hey, life is random too. The song list obviously reflects my generational bias, when I was hitting dance clubs. But let's admit the obvious: Music *was* better from the 1960s through the '80s. I also attach a bonus list of songs for deeper reflection. They draw heavily from the Celtic tradition, because of my Irish and Scottish roots. Music with this keening soulfulness transports me to places I've never been before, and yet I've always known.

And speaking of deep peace, I will leave you with yet another mantra I composed to help calm my overactive mind: "All these bees inside my head—a mental hive I always dread / I've got to learn to be more Zen / If not now, then tell me when."

FAST DANCES

"Not My Slave," Oingo Boingo

"Let's Dance," Chris Montez

"When You Were Mine," Prince

"What Is Love," Haddaway

"Deadly Valentine," Charlotte Gainsbourg

"Just Like Heaven," The Cure

"Love Is a Beautiful Thing," Al Green

"(I'm a) Road Runner," Junior Walker and the All Stars

"Dreams," The Cranberries

"Who Told You That," Mavis Staples

"Midnight," Yaz

"You Dropped a Bomb on Me," The Gap Band

"Uncertain Smile," The The

"L.E.S. Artistes," Santigold

"Slow Motion," Blondie

"Everybody Needs Someone to Love," Solomon Burke

"I Wish I Knew (How It Would Feel to Be Free),"
    Solomon Burke

"Ramblin' Gamblin' Man," The Bob Seger System

"Family Affair," Mary J. Blige

"I Touch Myself," Divinyls

"I Melt With You," Modern English

"Everyday Is Like Sunday," Morrissey

"Johnny Come Home," Fine Young Cannibals

"Rainin' in Paradize," Manu Chao

"Let's See Action," Pete Townshend

"Shoop," Salt-N-Pepa

"Goodbye to You," Scandal
"Fun," Sly and the Family Stone
"Story of My Life," Social Distortion
"De Musica Ligera," Soda Stereo
"Drinkee," Sofi Tukker
"Baby Baby," The Vibrators
"MaliAyiti," Vox Sambou
"To Lose My Life," White Lies
"Moving to the Left," Woods

SLOWER DANCES

"Stay With Me," Temptations
"Dance," Nas
"Forever Young," Alphaville
"Another Age," Robert Earl Thomas
"Un autre que moi," Fishbach
"Ghosts," V V Brown
"Head Hang Low," Julian Cope
"Hotter Colder," This Is the Kit
"Kiss," Prince
"Throw Your Arms Around Me," Hunters & Collectors
"Take Time to Know Her," Percy Sledge
"Fitxadu," Sara Tavares
"I Don't Know Why," Stevie Wonder
"Black Swan," Thom Yorke
"Hypnotized," Fleetwood Mac
"Big Bad Handsome Man," Imelda May

BONUS LIST

Songs for Meditation—About Life and Whatever Lies Beyond

———

"Meet on the Ledge," Fairport Convention

"Brightness in the Flame," Iain Matthews

"Dust," Fleetwood Mac

"Deep Peace," Donovan

"September Song," Lotte Lenya

"You Want It Darker," Leonard Cohen

"Beware of Darkness," George Harrison

"Within You Without You," The Beatles

"Don't Let Me Know," The Joy Formidable

"Hector the Hero," Natalie MacMaster and Donnell Leahy

"All Is Well," Ollabelle

"Bright Morning Star," Oysterband

"Into White," Cat Stevens

"All Kinds of Roses," Yusuf Islam

"With You in Mind," Marianne Faithfull

"Ghost Dance," Patti Smith

"Another Day," This Mortal Coil

"Wuthering Heights," Kate Bush

ACKNOWLEDGMENTS

Writing this book was part of my healing process, like learning to swallow, walk and speak clearly again. I never could have labored over my keyboard, with increasingly dexterous hands and mental clarity, if my reassembly had not been guided and inspired by many people. I give my love and gratitude to my wife, Camille, and our sons Joseph and Nathaniel, and to our extended family, especially Steve, Pippa, Cindy, Dave, Margaret, Art, Don, Sue, Caitlin, Julie, Ike and Lucy.

I will also forever hold dear in my heart the gracious and gifted staff of the stroke ward at the Davies Campus of California Pacific Medical Center in San Francisco, including Rebecca Reilly, Glenn-Clifford David Gangano, Jason Overcash, Eliano Oliveira, Nella Tay Bracken, Sarah Cook, Meaza Tesfamariam, Thomas Macasaet, Dr. Andy Knapp and Dr. Stephen Ng.

My care continued after my hospital release, and among those who helped me rejoin life outside were Dr. Michael Ke and rehabilitation specialists Gary Petersen, Vladislava Ryvkin, Janice Wong, Lily Murphy, Sonya Richardson, Jennifer Connolly and Linda Chu.

Many friends and neighbors also rushed to help me and my family when we needed them most, among them Ruth Henrich, Jane Wattenberg, Sam Chase, Connie Matthiessen, Mark Schapiro, Gary Kamiya, Louise Rubacky, Cheryl Nardi, Qunicy McCoy, Carla Sorey-Reed, Marianne Bachers, Rafael Trujillo, Margaret Weir and Linda and Jim Khatami.

I must also thank the progressive leaders and activists of San Francisco, who kept me in my city's political loop and trusted that I would regain my public voice, especially Jane Kim, David Campos, Hillary Ronen, Tom Ammiano, Tim Redmond, Jeff Kositsky and Jon Golinger.

And I want to express my deep appreciation to Chronicle Books chairman Nion McEvoy and to publisher Mark Tauber—creator of Prism, the new Chronicle Books imprint—for recognizing there was a book in my outpouring of online introspection; to Chronicle Books executive editor Cara Bedick for her skilled and sensitive craft; and to copyeditor Elsa Dixler for her nuanced final polish.

Finally, I thank Karen Croft, who—as always—worked as my production partner on this project.

If I have failed to recall any other important names, please forgive my mental lapse. After all . . . *I had a fucking stroke!*

The cover art by the ecstatic William Blake came to me, as if in a vision, in the middle of my stroke. While suffering my brain trauma—but still strangely oblivious to what was happening to me—I posted a grand, puzzling Facebook message about the human predicament. I ended by quoting a famous proverb from Blake's 1793 book *The Marriage of Heaven and Hell*: "If the doors of perception were cleansed every thing would appear to man as it is, Infinite." And I attached an illustration from Blake's book, showing a man in the throes of either agony or ecstasy—or both. Much later, while writing this memoir, I knew that its cover had to feature a hallucinatory art piece from Blake's illustrated book of poetry and prose. Blake possessed a rare understanding that heaven and hell were not polar opposites, but together formed a unified whole. Human existence in fact thrived on this tension between torment and transcendence. "Without Contraries is no progression," wrote Blake. This is the way I felt after my stroke had done its worst to me. I was ravaged, and reborn, all at once.

In memory of Paula and Lyle Talbot,
and all those who lived life fully
and brought joy to others

"Paths that cross will cross again."
PATTI SMITH